THE SIRTFOOD DIET

Beginner's cookbook with easy and healthy recipes to activate your skinny gene and burn fat. This book will help you to lose weight fast and improve your life

JENNIFER MATTEN

DISCLAIMER

All intellect contained in this book is given for enlightening and instructive purposes as it were. The creator isn't in any capacity responsible for any outcomes or results that radiate from the use of this material. Worthwhile endeavours have been made to give data that is both precise and viable. However, the creator isn't headed for the exactness or use/misuse of this data.

TABLE OF CONTENTS

INTRODUCTION 1

    1st phase menu 4

CHAPTER 1: SIRTFOOD DIET THEORY...........................**8**

    Task of the sirtuins in the body 10

    Is it healthy and long-lasting? 12

    These foods are allowed 14

CHAPTER 2: WHAT IS THE SKINNY GENE? **16**

CHAPTER 3: THE SCIENTIFIC BASIS OF SIRT DIET........**24**

    Who is the diet suitable for? 25

CHAPTER 4: DIET SIRT AND FAT **27**

CHAPTER 5: DIET SIRT AND PHYSICAL EXERCISE........**36**

CHAPTER 6: SIRT FOODS IN DETAIL **39**

CHAPTER 7: FOOD PLAN OF THE FIRST 7 DAYS **55**

    (DAY 1)... 55

    BREAKFAST... 55

        Green Juice (1 -2 servings)................................. 55

    LUNCH... 57

        Chicken Stir-Fry (1 serving)............................... 57

    DINNER..58

        Green Juice. Use the same recipe as above. 58

    (DAY 2).. 59

    BREAKFAST... 59

        Berry Juice (1 -2 servings) 59

    LUNCH...60

        Tuna Salad (1 serving).......................................60

DINNER 60

    Berry Juice. Use the same recipe as above. 60

(DAY 2) 61

BREAKFAST 61

    Berry Juice (1 -2 servings) 61

LUNCH 62

    Tuna Salad (1 serving) 62

DINNER 63

    Berry Juice. Use the same recipe as above. 63

(DAY 3) 64

BREAKFAST 64

    Green Juice with Blueberries (1 serving) 64

LUNCH 65

    Tofu-Veggie Stir-Fry (1-2 servings) 65

DINNER 66

    Green Juice with Blueberries. Follow the recipe above. 66

(DAY 4) 67

BREAKFAST 67

    Sweet Green Juice (1 serving) 67

LUNCH 68

    Teriyaki Salmon (2 servings) 68

    Apple Walnut Salad (1-2 servings) 70

DINNER 71

    Teriyaki Salmon 71

(DAY 5) 72

BREAKFAST 72

    Pita Pizza (1 serving) 72

LUNCH 73

    Refreshing Green Juice (1 serving) 73

DINNER 74

    Meat Loaf Pita Sandwich (1 servings) 74

(DAY 6) 75

BREAKFAST 75

    Soy Berry Smoothie (1 serving) 75

    Berry Yoghurt (1 serving) 75

LUNCH 76

    Lentil Curry (2 servings) 76

DINNER 78

    Lentil Curry 78

(DAY 7) 79

BREAKFAST 79

    Sweet Green Juice (1 serving) 79

LUNCH 80

    Teriyaki Salmon (2 servings) 80

    Apple Walnut Salad (1-2 servings) 81

DINNER 83

Teriyaki Salmon 83

CHAPTER 8: MAINTAINING **84**

CHAPTER 9: SHOPPING LIST **87**

Chapter 10: Recipes **91**

An apple and an egg 91

Sweet potato salad with bacon 92

Salad with melon and ham 93

Paleo Chicken Wraps 94

Chocolate Breakfast Muffins 95

Apple Cinnamon Wraps 96

Avocado and salmon salad buffet 97

Paleo-force bars 98

Vinaigrette 99

Spicy Ras-el-Hanout dressing 100

Chicken rolls with pesto 101

Mustard 102

Vegetarian curry from the crock pot: 103

Fried cauliflower rice: 104

Mediterranean paleo pizza: 106

Fried chicken and broccolini : 108

Braised leek with pine nuts: 109

Sweet and sour pan with cashew nuts: 110

Casserole with spinach and eggplant 111

Vegetarian paleo ratatouille: 112

Courgette and broccoli soup: 113

Frittata with spring onions and asparagus: 114

Cucumber salad with lime and coriander 115

Mexican bell pepper filled with egg: 116

Honey mustard dressing 117

Paleo chocolate wraps with fruits 118

Chocolate sauce 119

Hot sauce 120

Paleo breakfast salad with egg 121

Caesar dressing 122

Basil dressing 123

Strawberry sauce 124

Fresh chicory salad: 125

Grilled vegetables and tomatoes 126

Steak salad 127

Zucchini salad with lemon chicken 129

Fresh salad with orange dressing.. 130

Tomato and avocado salad 131

Arugula with fruits and nuts.. 132

Spinach salad with green asparagus and salmon...........................133

Brunoise salad 134

Broccoli salad..135

Ganache squares: 136

Date candy 137

Paleo bars with dates and nuts 138

Banana strawberry milkshake:.. 139

Buns with chicken and cucumber 140

Hazelnut balls 141

Stuffed eggplants 142

Chicken teriyaki with cauliflower rice.. 144

Curry chicken with pumpkin spaghetti... 146

French style chicken thighs 148

Spicy ribs with roasted pumpkin.. 149

Roast beef with grilled vegetables 151

Vegan Thai green curry...152

Indian yellow curry 154

Sweet potato hash browns 155

Tuna salad in red chicory...156

Paleolicious smoothie bowl 157

Granola...158

Herby Paleo French fries with herbs and avocado dip 159

Salad with bacon, cranberries and apple 161

Strawberry popsicles with chocolate dip 163

Hawaii salad 164

Rainbow salad for lunch.. 165

Strawberry and coconut ice cream 166

Coffee Ice Cream.. 167

Banana dessert...168

Salad with roasted carrots...169

Salmon with capers and lemon.......................................170

Pasta salad..171

Pine and sunflower seed rolls 172

Spiced burger 174

Chicken skewers with cashew sauce.............................. 176

Vegetable skewers.. 177

Pork chops with orange and mustard glaze 178

Grilled sweet potato with coriander dressing...............179

Conclusion...180

INTRODUCTION

The Sirt Food Diet (also called Sirt or Sirtuin Diet) was developed by the English nutrition experts Aidan Goggins and Glen Matten and triggered a real hype around the world. Because the concept is not only based on scientific studies - you should also be able to lose up to three kilograms a week in a fairly relaxed manner, activate muscle building and improve the body's defenses. But let's start from the beginning: the diet revolves around "Sirtfoods" - this is a newly discovered group of foods that are not only rich in vitamins and minerals, but are also supposed to activate the "skinny gene" Sirtuin. The body switches to a kind of survival mode - fat reserves are burned and the cells also renew and repair themselves faster. This special process leads to the desired weight loss, problem areas melt, muscle mass is built up more effectively and the immune system gains strength. Sirtuins also protect the body against stress and slow down the aging process - the skin should shine through the regular consumption of sirtuin foods.

The Sirtfood diet was chosen by singer Adele to help her lose weight, and it worked: Adele lost no less than 45 kilos associating the regime to the practice of Pilates, according to British tabloids. But how to put together a menu of such a new diet, which still causes many doubts even among nutritionists, still studying its principles and effects? How to do to include it without risks in the routine? First, it is important to understand how it works. The regimen includes calorie restriction for a week, but it also recommends foods rich in antioxidants and that stimulate sirtuins, enzymes that contribute to improving the metabolism of even glucose and adipose tissue and that may be linked to longevity. It is with this proposal that the diet promises to promote weight loss. There is still not much scientific evidence to support it. Yet,

The diet is divided into three stages:

The first one lasts three days and involves the consumption of up to a thousand calories daily, with fiber intake, in addition to recipes such as green juice, which increases satiety;

In the second, up to 1,500 calories should be consumed daily for four days, keeping the fibers and green juice;

After these two moments, the maintenance stage is entered, which does not define a caloric intake limit and starts to include more fresh foods. Once this process is completed, the creators of Sirtfood suggest to continue using the activators of sirtuins in the diet. Including, of course, fibers and green juice.

Nutritionist Renata Starling Torres, a specialist in nutrition in chronic non-communicable diseases, notes that a positive aspect of this plan is the presence of healthy foods that provide numerous health benefits, including stimulating the production of sirtuins. They are foods rich in antioxidants, which prevent the premature aging of cells that form free radicals. Among them, for example:

- Cabbage
- Arugula
- Parsley
- Capers
- Purple Onion
- Red and citrus fruits
- Date
- Turmeric
- Oilseeds
- Bitter chocolate

Nutritionist Renata Starling Torres, a specialist in nutrition in chronic non-communicable diseases, notes that a positive aspect of this plan is the presence of healthy foods that provide numerous health benefits, including stimulating the production of sirtuins. They are foods rich in antioxidants, which prevent the premature aging of cells that form free radicals. Among them, for example:

- Cabbage
- Arugula
- Parsley
- Capers
- Purple Onion
- Red and citrus fruits

- Date
- Turmeric
- Oilseeds
- Bitter chocolate

1st phase menu

(With a restriction of up to a thousand calories for three days)

Breakfast

1 scrambled egg OR omelet with saffron or turmeric and parsley, 1 cup of green tea.

Morning snack

1 glass of detox juice

Lunch

1 small piece of grilled or roasted salmon with capers, 1 dessert dish of kale salad, capers, red onion and lemon.

Afternoon snack

Mix of oilseeds: A Brazil nut, a walnut, two almonds and a hazelnut.

Dinner

1 grilled chicken fillet, 1 dessert plate of arugula salad with olive oil.

Evening snack

1 citrus fruit,
Chamomile tea.

2nd phase menu
(With a restriction of up to 1,500 calories for four days)

Breakfast

1 medium grilled tofu,
1 jar of nonfat plain yogurt.
Morning snack

1 glass of detox juice (recipe to follow).
Lunch

4 tablespoons of brown rice,
1 small bean scoop,
1 fillet of grilled or roasted saint-peter with capers,
1 dessert plate of cooked pumpkin.
Afternoon snack

5 dates,
2 squares of chocolate above 70% cocoa.

Dinner

4 tablespoons of grilled chicken baits,
1 dessert plate of arugula salad with olive oil.
Evening snack

1 citrus fruit,
Chamomile tea.

Maintenance menu
(To be included in the routine and generate food reeducation)

Breakfast

1 orange with pomace,
2 poached eggs,
1 Chestnut from Pará,
1 cup of chamomile tea.
Morning snack

1 glass of detox juice (recipe to follow).

Lunch

1/2 cooked sweet potato,
1 grilled tuna fillet with sesame,
1 dessert plate of sautéed spinach with red onion.

Afternoon snack

2 squares of chocolate above 70% cocoa.
Dinner

1 deep dish of tomato soup with mushrooms and basil.
Evening snack

1 citrus fruit,
Chamomile tea.

Detox Juice Recipe
(To be used always)

Yield: 3 servings

Ingredients:

2 large cups of green tea
2 kale leaves
1/2 large green apple
3 stalks of green celery with leaves
1 tablespoon of parsley
1/2 lemon juice
1/2 tablespoon green tea
3 tablespoons of grape
Method of preparation:

Beat all ingredients in a blender and consume without sweetening or straining.

CHAPTER 1:
SIRTFOOD DIET THEORY

Theoretically, this slimming diet is sold to make you lose weight quickly and without depriving yourself. It appeared for the first time in 2016 in a book soberly entitled The Sirtfood diet and written by two English graduates in nutritional medicine, Aidan Goggins and Glen Matten.

In practice, this involves consuming only "superfoods", rich in sirtuins, a family of enzymes that has 7 members (SIRT1, SIRT2... up to SIRT7). According to the authors, these enzymes with multiple benefits boost the immune system, protect against neurodegenerative diseases and act against cell aging.

Among the foods that would contain these famous enzymes are apples, blueberries, coffee, matcha tea, turmeric, dates, celery, onion, citrus, olive oil, arugula, soy but also... dark chocolate and red wine!

The Sirtuin Diet (in the original Sirtfood Diet) is based on proteins. But she still has nothing in common with Low-Carb, Paleo & Co. Because, as the name suggests, the focus is on a very special protein - the enzyme Sirtuin. Anyone who has thought directly of animal products when it comes to proteins is wrong.

They are plant foods that stimulate the formation of the enzyme and form the basic idea of the nutritional form. A new era of superfoods. And something else distinguishes the trend from all the others: long-term calories do not have to be counted, nor are certain foods prohibited.

The idea: inclusion instead of exclusion

The diet was developed by the British nutritionists Aidan Goggins and Glen Matten. Their theory: The enzyme, which is particularly active in lean people and fat loss, can be stimulated by eating certain foods.

Sirtuins are also released during fasting, but the inventors wanted to avoid the negative side effects of a strict fasting cure.

Kick start for the metabolism

At the beginning, a 2-phase diet is recommended to fuel the metabolism and the sirtuins. 1000 calories are consumed in the first 3 days. After that, the intake is increased to 1500 calories. Here you stick to green juices and sirtuin-based meals.

After 7 days you eat again as needed, of course still a potpourri of sirt foods. These phases are not a must! Even if you "only" integrate the sirt foods and live healthy, you will see success.

Task of the sirtuins in the body

The enzyme is responsible for cell protection in the body and thus also for defense against diseases, the aging process and the associated higher life expectancy. The fat metabolism is also significantly influenced by the sirtuins.

The creators of this diet claim that following the Sirtfood diet leads to rapid weight loss while maintaining muscle mass and protecting you from chronic illnesses.

Once you have completed your diet, we recommend that you continue to include sirtfoods foods and the green juice of your diet in your usual diet.

summary: the sirtfood diet is based on research into sirtuins, a group of proteins that regulate various body functions. some foods called sirtfoods can cause the body to produce more of these proteins.

Is it effective?

The authors of the Sirtfood diet make bold statements, including that the diet can overload weight loss, activate your "lean gene", and prevent disease.

The problem is that there is not much evidence to support them.

So far, there is no convincing evidence that the sirt food diet has a more beneficial effect on weight loss than any other low-calorie diet.

And although many of these foods have health benefits, long-term studies have not been conducted in humans to determine whether a diet rich in sirt foods has tangible health benefits.

Nevertheless, the book Sirtfood Diet presents the results of a pilot study that was carried out by the authors and in which 39 participants from their fitness center participated. However, the results of this study do not appear to have been published anywhere else.

For a week, the participants followed the diet and exercised daily. At the end of the week, participants lost an average of 3.2 kg and maintained or even gained muscle mass.

However, these results are hardly surprising. Limiting your calorie intake to 1,000 calories while exercising will almost always result in weight loss.

However, this type of rapid weight loss is neither authentic nor sustainable, and this study did not follow participants after the first week to determine whether they had gained weight, which is usually the case.

When your body is deprived of energy, in addition to burning fat and muscles, it also uses up its emergency energy reserves or glycogens.

Each glycogen molecule requires the storage of 3 to 4 water molecules. If your body uses glycogen, it will get rid of that water too. It's called "weight of water".

During the first week of extreme calorie reduction, only about a third of the weight loss came from fat, while the remaining two thirds came from water, muscles and glycogen.

As soon as your calorie intake increases, your body replenishes its glycogen stores and the weight returns immediately.

Unfortunately, this type of calorie restriction can also cause your body to lower its metabolism, forcing you to eat fewer calories a day than before.

This diet is likely to help you lose a few pounds first, but it will likely come back once the diet is over.

In terms of disease prevention, three weeks is probably not enough to have measurable long-term effects.

On the other hand, adding sirt foods to your usual long-term diet can be a good idea. In this case, however, you can skip the diet and start immediately.

Is it healthy and long-lasting?

Sirtfoods are almost all healthy products and can even have health benefits due to their antioxidant or anti-inflammatory properties.

However, if you eat only a few particularly healthy foods, you cannot satisfy all of your body's nutritional needs.

The Sirtfood plan is unnecessarily restrictive and has no net and unique health benefits over other types of plans.

In addition, it is generally discouraged to consume only 1000 calories without medical supervision. Even eating 1,500 calories a day is overly restrictive for many people.

The diet also requires drinking up to three green fruit juices a day. Although juices can be a good source of vitamins and minerals, they are also a source of sugar and contain almost no healthy fiber like whole fruits and vegetables (13).

In addition, drinking fruit juice all day for blood sugar and teeth is a bad idea (14).

Because the calorie and food choices in the diet are so limited, it is most likely lacking in protein, vitamins and minerals, especially in the first phase.

Due to the low-calorie content and restrictive eating habits, it can be difficult to follow this diet for the entire three weeks.

Add to this the high initial cost of buying a juicer, the book, and some rare and expensive ingredients, as well as the cost of preparing certain meals and juices, and this diet becomes impossible and unsustainable. for many people.

These foods are allowed

The British diet trend revolves around foods that are supposed to activate the valuable sirtuin enzymes through the plant substances they contain - without starving or counting calories. These include the following foods:

- Red onions
- walnuts
- garlic
- Blueberries and strawberries
- apples
- arugula
- Kale
- celery
- Spices like chili and turmeric
- Green tea
- red wine
- Dark chocolate (85% cocoa content)

The best? We can actually indulge in a glass of red wine or snack on chocolate in between, without a guilty conscience. The reason: red wine, especially Pinot Noir, contains the vegetable substance resveratrol, which is supposed to activate the miraculous sirtuins in the body. But of course, the rule applies to these delicacies as always: Please only enjoy in moderation! During the diet, which is carried out for at least a week, you should not exceed the limit of 1,500 calories a day. In order to achieve even better results, the test study found that the first three diet days were limited to just 1,000 calories. Regular exercise sessions are also recommended to build more muscle and quickly define the body.

CHAPTER 2:
WHAT IS THE SKINNY GENE?

Fasting-based diets have become very popular over the past few years. In fact, studies show that by fasting - that is, with moderate daily calorie restriction or by practicing a more radical, but less frequent intermittent fast - you can expect to lose about six pounds in six months and substantially reduce the risk of contracting certain diseases.

When we fast, the reduction of energy reserves activates the so-called "lean gene", which causes several positive changes. The accumulation of fat stops and the body blocks normal growth processes and enters "survival" mode. Fats are burned faster and the genes that repair and rejuvenate cells are activated. As a result, we lose weight and increase our resistance to disease.

The mysteries of thinness

Many studies have looked at the genetic specificities of overweight or obese people, Sadaf Farooqi, professor at the University of Cambridge, has chosen to focus on those of thin people. For this research, Sadaf Farroqi and his team worked with 1,622 thin volunteers, and used data from 1,985 severely obese people and 10,433 people of normal weight. Their DNA was collected and they answered a questionnaire on their state of health and their lifestyle.

Slimming is linked to genetics

The DNA study confirmed the results of previous studies: certain genes have a role in the risk of obesity and have allowed new discoveries to be made, in particular that other genes seem to be involved in slimming. The researchers gathered the data collected to develop a genetic risk index. "As we imagined, we found that obese people have a higher genetic risk index than people with normal weight," said one of the study authors. Conversely, thin people have a lower genetic risk index. 74% of the slim people in the study had slim and healthy people in their genealogy.

Target these genes to avoid obesity

"It's easy to make hasty judgments and criticize people for their weight, but science shows that things are much more complex, says Sadaf Farooqi. We have much less control over our weight than we would like". He now wants to push his research to identify precisely which gene influences thinness, this could help put the weight of specific treatment strategies for overweight people.

All this, however, has a price. Lower energy intake leads to hunger, irritability, exhaustion and loss of muscle mass. And the problem is precisely this with fasting-based diets: when they are followed correctly, they work, but they make us feel so bad that we cannot respect them. The question, then, is the following: is it possible to obtain the same results without having to impose that drastic drop in calories and, therefore, without suffering the negative consequences?

At this point we just have to present you the Sirt foods, a group of newly discovered foods. Sirt foods are particularly rich in special nutrients, capable of activating the same genes of thinness stimulated by fasting. These genes are sirtuins. They became famous thanks to an important study conducted in 2003, during which scientists analyzed a particular substance, resveratrol, present in the peel of black grapes, red wine and yeast, which would produce the same effects of calorie restriction without need to decrease energy intake. The researchers later found that other substances in red wine had a similar effect, which would explain the benefits of consuming this drink and why those who consume it get less fat.

This naturally stimulated the search for other foods containing a high concentration of these nutrients, capable of producing such a beneficial effect on the body, and studies gradually discovered several. If some are almost unknown, such as lovage, an herb that is by now very little used in cooking, the great majority is represented by well-known and widely used foods, such as extra virgin olive oil, red onions, parsley, chilli, curly kale, strawberries, capers, tofu, cocoa, green tea and even coffee.

The super regulators of metabolism

After the discovery of 2003, enthusiasm for the benefits of Sirt food skyrocketed. Studies reveal that these foods don't just mimic the effects of calorie restriction. They also act as super regulators of the entire metabolism, and burn fat, increase muscle mass and improve the health of the cells. The world of medical research was close to the most important nutritional discovery of the century. Unfortunately, a mistake was made: the pharmaceutical industry invested hundreds of millions of pounds in an attempt to turn Sirt foods into a sort of miracle pill, and the diet took a back seat. We do not share a similar pharmaceutical approach, which seeks (so far without result) to concentrate the benefits of these complex nutrients of plant origin into a single drug. Instead of waiting for the pharmaceutical industry to transform the nutrients of the foods we eat into a miraculous product (which may not work anyway), we find it more sensible to eat these substances in their natural form, that of foods, to take full advantage of them. This is the basis of our pilot experiment, with which we intended to create a diet containing the richest sources of Sirt foods and observe their effects.

A point in common among the healthiest diets in the world

During our studies we have discovered that the best Sirt foods are regularly consumed by the peoples who boast the lowest incidence of disease and obesity in the world.

Among the Kuna Indians, in the American continent, who seem immune from hypertension and with very low levels of obesity, diabetes, cancer and early death thanks to the intake of cocoa, excellent Sirt food, as well as in Okinawa, Japan, where a Sirt food, dry physique and longevity go hand in hand. In India, the passion for spicy foods, especially turmeric, gives good results in the fight against cancer. And in the traditional Mediterranean diet, which the rest of the western world envies, obesity is contained, and chronic diseases are the exception, not the norm. Extra virgin olive oil, wild green leafy vegetables, dried fruit, berries, red wine, dates and aromatic herbs are all effective Sirt foods, and they are all present in the Mediterranean diet.

Although Sirt foods are not a mainstay of nutrition in England today, the situation was quite different in the past. They were a basic element, and if many have become rare and others have even disappeared, we will soon see that it is possible to reverse the course.

For the first time, researchers have just highlighted a genetic cause of pathological thinness, associated with a risk of high mortality.

These studies, which point to the role of excess genes in underweight people who have difficulty eating, are published on Wednesday by the British scientific journal Nature.

The study, which involved 100,000 people, was led by Philippe Froguel (Imperial College / London and Institute Pasteur de Lille / France) and the Swiss team of Jacques Beckmann (University of Lausanne).

A fragment of chromosome 16 is known to be sometimes subject to fluctuations in the number of copies of its genes. The vast majority of people have two copies of each gene in this part of the chromosome, one transmitted by the mother, the other by the father. But about one in 2,500 people has only one copy (an under-dosage) and one in 2,000 has three copies (overdose of genes).

The Franco-Anglo-Swiss team had discovered in 2010 that the presence of a hole (a single copy) in this fragment of chromosome 16 could explain 1% of severe obesity.

It now demonstrates that people with an excess of genetic material (a "duplication") and therefore having three copies of this part of chromosome 16 have significant, even extreme thinness. They are up to 20 times more likely to be underweight than the general population.

These excess genes, 28 in number, are probably "appetite genes", underlines Professor Froguel.

Thus, in children, half of the carriers of this anomaly are underweight and find it very difficult to eat. They can suffer from a developmental disorder and weigh at 4 years the weight of a child of a year and a half, said AFP Professor Froguel.

The researchers identified 138 carriers of the anomaly out of the 100,000 people studied. "In a third of the cases, this mutation was absent in the parents and in the remaining two thirds it was hereditary," notes Professor Froguel.

Example of female thinness: 1m60 for 40 kg (BMI of the order of 15). In adults of both sexes, "at 40 kg mortality is as high as in people who weigh 100 kg," he says. This genetic defect affects longevity: "There is no old man" in identified carriers.

The excess or deficiency of certain genes on the same fragment of chromosome leads to opposite pathological consequences, underweight or obesity. It remains to clarify the mechanisms involved.

Of the 100,000 people studied, the researchers identified 138 carriers of the anomaly. "In a third of the cases, this mutation was absent in the parents and in the remaining two thirds it was hereditary," notes Professor Froguel. The region of chromosome 16 concerned by this duplication phenomenon comprising 28 genes, the next step will be to identify which one has an impact on appetite and weight. It could be a single gene or a combination of several of them.

This work also demonstrates that if certain genes from the same genetic region are present in excess (three copies) or deficiently (only one copy), this can lead, by a "mirror effect", to reverse pathological consequences - here the underweight or obesity.

CHAPTER 3:
THE SCIENTIFIC BASIS OF SIRT DIET

The main scientific evidence supporting this diet was the discovery that sirts foods are found in the diet of people with the lowest incidence of disease and obesity rates in the world, such as the American Kuna Indians or the Japanese of Okinawa.

However, much of the weight lost comes, not exactly from the food eaten, but from the drastic cut in energy value, particularly in the first phase. Due to the restriction and the juice-based diet, the loss of water and even loss of muscle mass causes the values on the scale to decrease substantially.

In addition, the studies were carried out in people whose physical activity is high, an activity that, in itself, activates the "lean genes" and contributes to the increase in longevity.

The traditional Mediterranean diet is the one that brings together the most consensus for weight loss and health improvement, being a dietary pattern that includes several sirts foods, such as virgin olive oil or red wine, fruit, vegetables, among others that contain vitamins and antioxidants.

IN SHORT...

It is useful to know the sirts foods that activate sirtuin since they are healthy foods and rich in antioxidants, which enhance health and can stimulate basal metabolism.

However, the majority of weight loss will be derived from the promoted energy restriction, which is the main factor for weight loss in any diet.

The Sirtfood diet is rich in healthy foods, but not healthy eating patterns. In addition to promoting rapid weight loss without elucidating what is being lost, quite serious health claims are made without any scientific evidence to support them.

Adding SIRT-rich foods to the food day is not at all a bad idea and can bring health benefits, but this is just another restrictive diet like so many others, with nothing special worth the buzz created around it.

Who is the diet suitable for?

The Sirtfood Diet is suitable for:

People with perseverance and discipline

nutrition-loving people with background knowledge

The Sirtfood Diet is not suitable for:

People who have a hard time consuming only a few calories every day

Smart tips for everyday life

Many advisers reveal which other foods are suitable for the sirt food diet and which other foods are combined with them. These can be helpful in order to better plan daily food preparation and thus make it easier. Because a comprehensive knowledge of sirtuins, their effects and how to best integrate them into your daily diet increases your stamina.

Relaxation is also an essential part of the sirt food diet. In stressful situations, the hormone cortisol is released, which, together with insulin, stimulates blood sugar levels and causes the body to feel hungry during periods of rest. Mainly due to the calorie reduction, one should avoid stressful situations in everyday life as much as possible. Small activities to balance out like a little walk in the fresh air can work wonders.

CHAPTER 4:
DIET SIRT AND FAT

The latest slimming trend is called Sirt Diet. A diet that is healthy and balanced and that promises important results in a short time by activating the genes of thinness naturally present in everyone. Conceived by British nutritionists Aiden Goggins and Matten Glen, who explained the mechanisms in a book, it is very popular among British celebrities who, following the example of the Dirt Diet, can today show off enviable lines. First of all, the singer Adele, who has lost 30 kilos, and Pippa Middleton. Revolutionary discovery or yet another fashion? The opinions on Sirt Diet are as always discordant, but we try to make things clear.

The key word for this new weight loss diet is sirtuins. Sirtuins are a family of genes responsible for lipolysis, our mood and strongly linked to longevity. By introducing the right foods into our bodies, these genes are activated and with their activation there is an acceleration of the metabolism and consequently a loss of weight. It is no coincidence that this diet is also called the lean gene. The foods to be introduced into the Sirt Diet are, for example, meat, fish, kale, chocolate, red wine, olive oil. It is not necessary to reduce the portion quantities, on the contrary, the results are obtained by eating abundantly.

The fat deposits on the body sometimes grow faster than we would like. Only: Fasting alone doesn't get them away. There is only one way to get rid of the excess energy: more exercise.

There are many ways to lose weight - unfortunately most diets leave us hungry and unsatisfied. If you don't have a lot of stamina, you will quickly let yourself be guided by hunger and throw your weight loss plans into the pile.

All you have to do to lose weight quickly is to follow the three rules below.

Rule 1: Eat less sugar and starch
The most important thing is to eat less sugar and starch (carbohydrates). Food with these ingredients has a huge impact on your insulin balance. Because, if you didn't know it already: the hormone insulin is the largest fat store in our body.

So, if we lower the insulin level through a low-carbohydrate diet, the fat has more time to get out of the fat stores and the body begins to burn these fats instead of carbohydrates.

Another benefit of low insulin level is that the kidneys flush excess sodium and water out of the body. This not only reduces flatulence, but also water retention.

If you follow this tip, you can lose up to five kilos of body fat and water in a week - sometimes even more!

The women who were on a low carb diet ate until they felt full. The participants in the low-fat diet ate reduced calories and often remained hungry.

Therefore: cut out carbohydrates, lower your insulin level and you will automatically start eating less. The fat burning then starts all by itself!

Conclusion: Eating less sugar and carbohydrates will lower your insulin levels and curb your appetite, so you can lose weight without starving yourself.

Rule 2: Eat more protein, fat, and vegetables

All of your meals should contain at least one source of protein and fat and be served with low-carb vegetables. If you follow this rule, you will automatically eat the recommended amount of carbohydrates - namely 20 to 50 grams per day.

High protein foods:

Meat: beef, chicken, pork, lamb, bacon, etc.

Fish & seafood: salmon, trout, shrimp, lobster, etc.

Eggs: Eggs enriched with omega-3 fatty acids or free-range ones are best

The importance of proteins cannot be emphasized enough. Because just consuming them burns your metabolism by up to 80 to 100 more calories a day.

High protein diets can also help you think about eating up to 60 percent less. It also helps to reduce the desire for a midnight snack and makes you so full that you automatically eat 441 fewer calories a day.

When it comes to losing weight, protein is the king of nutrients!

The best low-carb vegetables:

- broccoli
- cauliflower
- spinach
- (Kale
- Brussels sprouts
- chard
- salad
- cucumber
- celery

You can eat as much of these vegetables as you want without a guilty conscience. Because no matter how much of it you eat, you will never consume more than 20-50 grams of carbohydrates a day.

A meat and vegetable diet contain all the fiber, vitamins and minerals you need to live a healthy life. So, there is no physiological need for grain!

Eat two to three times a day. If you are still hungry in the evening, have a fourth meal.

The best sources of fat:

- olive oil
- coconut oil
- avocado oil
- butter
- lard

The best fat for cooking is coconut oil. It is high in fats known as medium chain triglycerides (MCTs). These fats are healthier than others and can better boost your metabolism.

Don't be afraid to use these fats just because they are fats. You should never go on a low carb and low-fat diet at the same time. Because you would definitely feel bad and that jeopardizes the success of the weight loss.

There is also no reason to avoid these healthy fats. Because studies show that - contrary to popular belief - saturated fatty acids do not increase the risk of heart disease.

Conclusion: Every meal should consist of a protein source, a fat source and a low-carb vegetable. This automatically moves you in the desired 20-50 gram carbohydrate range, which lowers your insulin level.

Rule 3: Exercise three times a week

You don't have to do competitive sports to lose weight with this diet, but exercise helps your body lose fat and, above all, stay tight.

It is best to exercise three to four times a week. When you go (or want to) to the gym, a combination of conscientious warm-up, strength training, and stretching exercises is perfect.

If you train with weights, you burn calories and keep your metabolism busy, which in turn helps you lose weight. Studies have shown that you can even build muscle while losing a lot of body fat.

If you are not the "gym freak", you can of course do cardio workouts and keep fit with swimming, running or walking.

Conclusion: Do best strength training. If that's not your thing, you can do cardio training.

Optional: insert a cheat day

If you want, you can introduce a cheat day every week where you eat a little more carbohydrates. A day on the weekend is best for this.

It is important that you do not overdo it on this day, but instead use healthy carbohydrates, which can be found in rice, quinoa, potatoes and fruits, for example. In addition, your Cheat Day should not become Cheat Week - otherwise you will not see any success.

Of course, you don't have to start a day like this, but the increased carbohydrate intake can have a positive effect, since it stimulates fat-burning hormones. So, don't worry if you weigh a little more after your cheat day, most of it is water, which you will lose again in the following days.

Conclusion: Eating a little more carbohydrates one day a week is absolutely fine, if not absolutely necessary.

Do I have to count calories and proteins?

The answer is simple: no. As long as you eat low carbohydrates and eat a lot of protein, fat and vegetables, you do not have to pay attention to a certain number of calories.

Of course, if it's important to you, you can still count how many calories you eat. There are special apps that help you count.

The goal of this diet is to eat less than 20-50 grams of carbohydrates a day. The remaining calories consist of proteins and healthy fat.

How much will I lose weight on this diet?

If you follow all three rules, you can lose up to five kilos in the first week. After that you will lose weight continuously. Since everybody reacts differently to the change in diet, these figures are only to be understood as a guide.

If this is your first diet, you will see results very quickly. It also depends on the initial weight. People who weigh more also lose weight faster and more.

You may feel a little strange in the first few days. Your body has spent most of its life processing carbohydrates. So, it may take some time for him to get used to burning fat now.

At the beginning of this change in diet, you may get a low-carb fever. The term describes a condition in which you feel flabby, irritable and constantly hungry and may also have a headache. These symptoms are caused by the absence of carbohydrates. The "fever" usually disappears after a few days. Sodium or hot broth can help in this initial phase.

As soon as your body gets used to the new circumstances, you will quickly and clearly feel better. You will be positive and energetic. At this point you are officially a "Fat Burning Monster".

In addition to weight loss, the low carb diet can bring you many other benefits:

- It lowers your blood sugar level
- It lowers your cholesterol level while the "good" cholesterol increases
- Your blood pressure will improve significantly

And best of all: Low carb diets are easier to hold out than low fat diets!

Conclusion: If you stick to the rules, your chances of losing a lot of weight are very good. However, how much you can lose weight varies from person to person. In addition, this low carb diet can also have a positive effect on your general health.

You don't have to go hungry to lose weight

If you have health problems or are taking medication, you should talk to your doctor before dieting.

By reducing carbohydrates and a lower insulin level, your hormone balance also changes, causing your body and your brain to "want" to lose weight.

This drastically reduces your hunger and appetite and you can hardly fail on the diet. So, you can lose two to three times as much as with classic diets.

Another benefit of this diet - especially for the impatient - is that the initial loss of water retention can make a big difference on the scales.

CHAPTER 5:
DIET SIRT AND PHYSICAL EXERCISE

Since 52% of Americans think it is easier to pay their taxes than to understand how to eat healthy, it is important to choose a diet that becomes a lifestyle rather than a single diet. For some of us, losing weight or maintaining a healthy weight is not that difficult, but the Sirtfood diet can help people in difficulty. But what about the combination of diet and exercise? Is it advisable to avoid exercise altogether or to introduce it once you have started the diet?

The SirtDiet principles

With around 650 million overweight adults around the world, it's important to find healthy foods and doable exercise programs, don't throw away everything you love, and don't have to exercise all the time. time. Week. The Sirtfood diet does just that: The idea is that certain foods activate the "lean gene" pathways that are usually activated by fasting and exercise. The good news is that some foods and drinks, including dark chocolate and red wine, contain chemicals called polyphenols that activate genes that mimic the effects of exercise and fasting.

Exercise for the first few weeks

During the first or second week of the diet, when your calorie intake is reduced, it makes sense to stop or reduce exercise while your body is adjusting to fewer calories. Listen to your body and do not exercise when you are tired or have less energy than usual. Instead, continue to focus on the principles that apply to a healthy lifestyle, such as: B.: A reasonable daily amount of fiber, protein, and fruits and vegetables.

As soon as the diet becomes a way of life

During exercise, it is important to ideally consume protein one hour after exercise. The protein repairs muscles after exercise, relieves pain and can promote regeneration. There are a variety of recipes that contain proteins perfect for post-workout consumption, e.g. For example: B. Sirt Chili con Carne or turmeric-chicken-kale salad. If you want something lighter, you can try the Sirt Blueberry smoothie and add protein powder for more benefits. The type of fitness you exercise is up to you. However, if you are training at home, you can choose when you want to exercise, what types of exercises are right for you, and are short and convenient.

The Sirtfood diet is a great way to change your eating habits, lose weight, and feel healthier. The first few weeks can be difficult, but it's important to check which foods are best to eat and which delicious recipes are right for you. Be kind to yourself for the first few weeks, as your body adapts and trains when you want to. If you are already exercising moderately or intensively, you may be able to continue as usual or manage your fitness based on the change in diet. As with any change in diet and exercise, it all depends on the person and how much effort you can make.

CHAPTER 6:
SIRT FOODS IN DETAIL

Stop restrictions, make way for a new feeding method. Here is Sirt food or the art of healthy eating, without depriving yourself.

It's a small revolution in the world of nutrition. Its name is already in everyone's mouths across the Channel: "The Sirt food diet" promises to convince the most resistant to diets. Because this one is not like the others. No question of depriving yourself, but rather of adding elements to your diet.

The principle is simple: bet everything on "superfoods", such as apples, onions, green tea … or dark chocolate and red wine. These are natural activators of the sirtuin enzymes present in our body, themselves endowed with the capacity to stimulate the "discomfort of thinness". Aidan Goggins and Glen Matten define themselves as " nutrition geeks ", and can boast of the support of British sportsmen and top models. Two years after their first book, "The health delusion", the duo are back to bring THE solution to weight disorders. Their diet would be able to make you lose 7 pounds in 7 days (about 3 kgs).

This diet comes from England, and, more precisely, from two nutritionists: Aidan Goggins and Glen Matten. Their objective? Eat healthy rather than lose weight at all costs, because, unlike other diets programmed to drastically lose weight, even unhealthy, the Sirt Food diet rather wants to stimulate the immune system, while eliminating fat. Besides, the Sirtfood diet would be able to make you lose 3 pounds in 7 days, without any deprivation.

By favoring sirt foods, this diet aims to improve your mode of consumption. Among these greedy "elected", there are many fruits and vegetables such as apples, citrus fruits, strawberries, kale but also parsley, red onion, capers, green tea, soy, turmeric, olive oil, coffee and, more surprisingly, red wine and chocolate (dark of course)! For the most suspicious, know that the countries where people eat the most sirt foods (Japan and Italy) are ranked among the healthiest in the world.

It authorizes the consumption

of foods that are prohibited in most other slimming diets, including, in particular, chocolate and red wine. If its creators are to be believed, it would allow, despite this, to lose up to 3 kg in the space of 7 days without really depriving yourself. Here we give you the typical menu for this diet which has already won over more than one.

The typical menu

Here is an example of a typical sirtfood day menu:

- At breakfast: soy yogurt mixed with berries, chopped nuts and dark chocolate. If you prefer to opt for salty, start the day with a bacon omelet accompanied by red chicory and parsley.

- At lunch: a sirtfood salad (chicory leaves, avocado, lovage, capers, etc.) will do the trick. But you can also replace it with a pita garnished with cheese, hummus and turkey.

- At dinner: sautéed shrimps with buckwheat noodles and kale. You can also opt for a homemade pizza made with sirtfood foods.

During the first 3 days of the diet, it is advisable to limit yourself to 1000 calories per day by drinking 3 green juices made from foods rich in sirtuins. From the 4th to the 7th day, the diet allows you to bring your daily caloric consumption to 1500 calories always by including in large quantities foods rich in sirtuins in the preparation of these meals.

This basically amounts to taking two sirtfood smoothies and two meals rich in sirtuins per day. Finally, from the 8th day, you must find a balanced daily diet while maintaining sirtfood in your meals.

Slimming without really depriving yourself with sirtuins

The sirtfood diet is based on the principle that, consuming foods rich in sirtuins is enough to lose weight without actually having to deprive yourself. Sirtuins are proteins naturally synthesized by the body, which increase the body's ability to burn fat, activate the metabolism and consolidate muscle mass. They also have an anti-aging effect.

They can be found in around twenty fairly common foods, including red wine, dark chocolate, apples, soy, dates, buckwheat, parsley, arugula, spinach, celery, capers, l olive oil, green tea, etc.

The sirtfood diet is very attractive, because it allows you to lose weight without suffering too much by adopting a French menu simple and easy to carry out. However, like all weight loss programs of this type, this diet presents relatively significant risks, especially if it is prolonged beyond the first 7 days.

WHAT TO EAT?

With the sirt food Diet, you don't have to pay attention to the contents of your basket or deprive yourself of delicious chocolate desserts to keep your figure. The principle of this slimming diet is simple: consume foods rich in sirtuins. Sirtuins are fat-burning enzymes that activate metabolism and help consolidate muscle mass. They are contained in foods such as:

- Chocolate
- The Red wine
- Extra virgin olive oil
- Nuts
- The celery
- Spinach
- Parsley
- The onions red
- Soy
- The strawberries
- Apples
- The blueberries
- The goji berries
- Dates
- Green tea
- Coffee.

Because of their richness in sirtuins, these foods, called superfoods, lead to rapid weight loss by removing excess fat, improve muscle performance and keep you on track for your health. Favoring them in your diet is therefore an effective way to shed those extra pounds and reshape your figure.

According to its two founders, the sirt food Diet would have the same effects as a sports activity, that is to say that it would burn the maximum amount of fat and strengthen physical health through the consumption of these super -food.

Very fashionable, the Sirtfood Diet has many followers including some celebrities like the British singer Adèle and the model Jodie Kidd. Lose weight quickly by consuming foods rich in sirtuins like chocolate, here is the idea behind this new slimming diet.

The sirt food Diet is the trend diet of the moment. He promises to lose 3 kg per week by consuming foods like chocolate and red wine.

Forces

If you adopt it, you would not need to do without gourmet chocolate recipes, even less to exclude this delicious food from your menus. This regime has indeed some advantages. At first, by choosing it, you will not have to deprive yourself of chocolate, wines or fats, so yes, the chocolate bars at 4 p.m. are allowed without any problem.

In addition, it allows those who want to lose a few inches of size to achieve this in a short period of time without subjecting themselves to dietary restrictions such as "ban sugar from their diet" or "avoid drinking wine ".

If you've always dreamed of a slimming diet where you could easily enjoy chocolate bars or indulge yourself with a good glass of red wine, the Sirtfood Diet method is the one for you.

plan, including kale, berries, ginger, turmeric, green tea, and olive oil. Here is an introduction to some of the top sirt foods - only enjoy them as part of a balanced diet with a variety of other healthy foods.

1. Chia seeds

In the world of sirt foods, chia seeds are considered to be moderately sirtuin inactivating foods, which the authors of the sirt food diet describe in their book as the equivalent of walking and getting into a food intensive sweating session in the gym.

Whether the claims contain water or not, there is no debate that chia seeds pack an incredible amount of nutrients in a small package, making them an efficient way to boost nutrient deficiencies like fiber (11 grams per ounce, or 44 percent of the daily value) and heart-healthy omega-3 fats (five grams per ounce). Chia is also a good source of vegetable protein. Simply sprinkle over a smoothie bowl, add to the smoothies or mix with oatmeal.

2. Cinnamon

In a study presented at the 2017 American Society for Biochemistry and Molecular Biology's annual meeting, researchers used a computer model to determine whether cinnamon activated Sirt-1 and found promising compounds. This is not proof yet, but an interesting building block for future research.

But cinnamon is still on the list of sirt foods because it contains strong polyphenols, herbal compounds with antioxidant and anti-inflammatory properties. And there are some research that suggests that cinnamon can help control blood sugar by slowing carb digestion and improving the body's response to insulin. It goes well with coffee, hot chocolate, cabbage, roasted pumpkin, soups, smoothies and spices for lean pork.

3. Cocoa

The suggested sirtuin-activating nutrient in cocoa is epicatechin, a powerful antioxidant that is also found in tea and grapes. In a 2016 animal study, cocoa increased Sirtuin-1, but keep in mind that the jump from mouse to human is a big one.

As a food rich in polyphenols, pure cocoa promotes healthy blood circulation, which is important for the supply of nutrients and oxygen as well as for general health. Remember that the benefits come from the cocoa plant and not from the addition of sugar, salt, and fat in processed candy bars. Look for the highest proportion chocolate you can find to get the greatest benefits.

4. Coffee

Coffee is the primary source of antioxidants in the U.S. diet. His sirt food creed comes from his polyphenol, caffeic acid. Animal studies with caffeic acid (and another antioxidant polyphenol in coffee, chlorogenic acid) showed that obese mice lost weight, including belly fat.

It also lowered insulin, triglyceride and cholesterol levels while increasing fatty acid oxidation and blocking the formation of new fat cells in the liver. While this study was done on mice rather than humans, the results suggest that coffee contains compounds that could theoretically help improve body weight and how well the body breaks down fat.

5. Olive oil

The suspected sirtuin-activating polyphenols in virgin olive oil are oleuropein and hydroxytyrosol. What we do know is that olive oil is a key component of the heart-healthy Mediterranean diet, which can also support a weight management plan.

It is rich in monounsaturated fats that improve cholesterol when it replaces saturated fats or refined carbohydrates. Extra virgin varieties have the most complex polyphenol profiles, although they decrease with air, heat and time. Many bottles have a harvest date so you can find the freshest olive oil.

6. Ginger

Ginger is a cousin of turmeric, which is also on the list of sirt foods. It contains gingerol, which has anti-inflammatory and antioxidant properties. It has long been used as a natural cure for motion sickness and can generally help with nausea and dizziness.

Fresh chopped ginger gives turkey burgers a high-contrast aroma. It is also a peppery and invigorating addition to smoothies and salad dressings. Fry it with other flavors like onions and garlic before adding vegetables for a quick weekly side dish. (Pro tip: use a spoon and some pressure to peel the gnarled skin slightly.)

7. Matcha

The well-known long-lived, healthy population groups of Japan may like something with their love for tea. Green tea is included as a staple food due to its antioxidant epigallocatechin gallate (EGCG). The authors of Sirtfood Diet particularly recommend the powdered Matcha green tea form.

Regardless of whether you prefer green, white, oolong, or black, tea drinkers tend to have lower bad LDL cholesterol and better HDL cholesterol. Regular tea also contains some caffeine for an extra boost. Enjoy it in smoothies or as a poaching liquid for cod - or just drink a cup as part of your morning ritual.

8. Raspberries

Raspberries and other berries such as strawberries and blackberries have adopted sirtuin-activating polyphenols. No wonder that berries are antioxidant superstars. Raspberries, especially quercetin and gallic acid, and strawberries are notable sources of fisetin. Fresh summer raspberries are great on their own and frozen raspberries can be enjoyed all year round in a deserted smoothie or an unexpectedly fresh salsa. Both are high in fiber and vitamin C.

9. Kale

Kohl's most important antioxidants in the sirt food diet are kaempferol and quercetin, which have been tested primarily in laboratories and animals for their anti-inflammatory effects. They are undoubtedly waging a radical struggle on your behalf.

And as if that wasn't enough, a cup of kale contains twice as much vitamin A and more vitamin C than an orange. Remove the stems, roll them and cut them crosswise into ribbons (chiffonade) before massaging them with your favorite dressing for a few minutes. Add these marinated kale ribbons and the fruits you have nearby to your favorite grain like Farro, Wheat Berry, Sorghum or Freekeh for a quick and healthy whole grain salad.

10. Red wine

Red wine has made a name for itself in health circles because it contains resveratrol, a polyphenol that can activate sirtuins. Human observational studies suggest that moderate intake could have health benefits for older adults, especially heart health, and possibly brain longevity and health.

As a traditional part of the Mediterranean diet, it is intended to be enjoyed with a reasonable amount of food (e.g. a 5 ounce glass for women per day). Of course, it is not for everyone and there are many other ways to eat and drink healthily for anyone who prefers to avoid wine for some reason.

11. Turmeric

Turmeric is the golden child of healthy food these days. It looks like ginger, but it's the color of sweet potatoes inside. Turmeric is a major ingredient in curry powders, and the active ingredient is curcumin, an anti-inflammatory and antioxidant compound. The body doesn't take it very well, so it's good that black pepper increases absorption by 2,000 percent.

If you enjoy it with some healthy fat, the body can also absorb this fat-soluble antioxidant better. Make your own "golden milk" by whisking almond milk, coconut milk, turmeric, black pepper, ginger and honey (optional) on low heat. Sprinkle cinnamon over it and enjoy.

12. Medjool appointments

The Sirtfood Diet does not tolerate added sugar, but Medjool dates that contain the polyphenols gallic acid and caffeic acid are permitted. A 2011 study published in the Journal of Nutrition found that eating dates did not significantly increase blood sugar and was even associated with lower rates of diabetes and heart disease.

If you throw back four dates, you have reached 30 percent of your daily fiber intake. They are also a good source of potassium, a nutritional deficiency in the American diet that helps with hydration, muscle contraction and carbohydrate metabolism. If you've kept your taste buds from overly sweet flavors, you may want to cut some dates into pieces and sparingly add them to savory dishes like curries, cereal salads, and pan sauces for fried chicken.

13. Capers

Capers boast powerful anti-inflammatory effects, offering a cocktail of vitamins, minerals, and antioxidants. They have only 23 calories per 100 grams, and provide large amounts of calcium, potassium, vitamin K, riboflavin, iron, copper, and phytonutrients. Quercentin and rutin, the key antioxidants in capers, have strong analgesic, antibacterial, and anti-carcinogenic properties. Rutin helps prevent and treat hemorrhoids, improves circulation, and reduces bad cholesterol levels in obese patients. Quercentin inhibits tumor growth and boosts immune function. The best way to use capers is adding them to salads, pasta, and casseroles.

CHAPTER 7

FOOD PLAN OF THE FIRST 7 DAYS

(DAY 1)
BREAKFAST

(ALSO SUITABLE FOR MID-MORNING SNACK OR AFTERNOON TEA)

Green Juice (1 -2 servings)

Ingredients

- 75g Kale
- 30 g arugula
- 10 g parsley
- 150 g celery
- medium green apple
- lemon
- ½ teaspoon matcha green tea
- tablespoon agave or natural honey (optional)

Method:

1. Clean the vegetables and fruit. Put the kale, arugula and parsley in the juicier or blender. Add some water if you are using a blender.

2. Next, Juice the celery and apple.

3. Squeeze the lemon into the resulting juice above.

4. Use a fine mesh strainer to strain the juice it you like. This is optional.

5. Pour some juice into a glass and add the matcha green tea. Stir to dissolve completely. Then top up with the rest of the juice. If using a blender, add the green tea into the blender and blitz foe a few second.

6. You may add some water to the green juice before drinking.

LUNCH

Chicken Stir-Fry (1 serving)

Ingredients:

- 1 boneless and skinless chicken breast (about 120 g, sliced thinly)
- 50 g buckwheat or buckwheat noodle (soba)
- 100 g kale (cleaned and chopped)
- 1 small red onion (peeled and chopped)
- 1 clove garlic (peeled and chopped)
- ½ inch ginger root (peeled and sliced)
- 1 teaspoon turmeric
- Some parsley (as a garnish)
- 1 or more bird's eye chilli (optional)
- ½ lemon (optional)
- 1-2 tablespoon extra-virgin olive oil Seasonings: salt, pepper, sesame oil, soy sauce or tamari sauce, oyster Sauce, etc.

Method:

1. Marinate the chicken with the turmeric powder and some salt. Pepper and soy sauce. Just add a bit of the seasonings as you will adjust the taste again later.

2. Cook the buckwheat/ buckwheat noodle according to the packet instructions.

3. Heat a large work or frying pan. Add the kale with some sale water. Cook it for a few minutes until it wilts. Take it out and cool under running water to keep the color.

4. Dry the wok or pan and heat up the olive oil. Add the red onion, garlic and ginger. Stir fry for a few minutes.

5. Add the chicken and the chili Into the wok. Cook them until brown or done.

6. Add some water to create some sauce or gravy (add more to get a nice gravy). Bring the mixture to a simmer. Adjust the taste again by adding some seasonings like soy sauce, sesame oil, oyster sauce, etc.

7. Add in the kale. If you are using buckwheat noodle, you can also add the noodles to the chicken mixture. Coat everything with thee sauce.

8. Take out and garnish with the chopped parsley. Squeeze the lemon if using.

DINNER

Green Juice. Use the same recipe as above.

(DAY 2)
BREAKFAST

(ALSO SUITABLE FOR MID-MORNING SNACK OR AFTERNOON TEA)

Berry Juice (1 -2 servings)

Ingredients:

- 1 cup strawberries
- 1 cup blueberries
- 1 green apple (cored and cut)
- 50 g celery
- 1-2 stalks parsley
- ½ lemon
- ½ teaspoon matcha green tea

Method:

1. Clean the vegetables and fruit. Juice or blend the fruits and vegetables.
2. Squeeze the lemon into the resulting juice above.
3. Use a fine mesh strainer to strain the juice if you like. This is optional.
4. Pour some juice into a glass and add the matcha green tea. Stir to dissolve completely. Then top up with the rest of the juice. If using a blender, add the green tea into the blender and blitz for a few seconds.
5. You may add some water to dilute the juice before drinking.

LUNCH

Tuna Salad (1 serving)

Ingredients:

- ½ of a can of tuna (tuna in brine/water or oil)
- 1 small red onion (peeled and chopped)
- 50 g arugula/rocket (more or less to your liking)
- 50 g red chicory (more or less to your liking)
- 2 medjool dates (pitted and chopped)
- 30 g celery (chopped or sliced
- 1-2 stalks parsley (chopped)
- 1 tablespoon capers
- 1 tablespoon extra-virgin olive oil
- 1 tablespoon lemon juice
- Salt& pepper

Method:

1. Drain and flake the tuna. Clean and chopped the vegetables.

2. Mix all the ingredients in a large salad bowl. Enjoy.

DINNER

Berry Juice. Use the same recipe as above.

(DAY 2)

BREAKFAST

(ALSO SUITABLE FOR MID-MORNING SNACK OR AFTERNOON TEA)

Berry Juice (1 -2 servings)

Ingredients:

- 1 cup strawberries
- 1 cup blueberries
- 1 green apple (cored and cut)
- 50 g celery
- 1-2 stalks parsley
- ½ lemon
- ½ teaspoon matcha green tea

Method:

6. Clean the vegetables and fruit. Juice or blend the fruits and vegetables.
7. Squeeze the lemon into the resulting juice above.
8. Use a fine mesh strainer to strain the juice if you like. This is optional.
9. Pour some juice into a glass and add the matcha green tea. Stir to dissolve completely. Then top up with the rest of the juice. If using a blender, add the green tea into the blender and blitz for a few seconds.
10. You may add some water to dilute the juice before drinking.

LUNCH

Tuna Salad (1 serving)

Ingredients:

- ½ of a can of tuna (tuna in brine/water or oil)
- 1 small red onion (peeled and chopped)
- 50 g arugula/rocket (more or less to your liking)
- 50 g red chicory (more or less to your liking)
- 2 medjool dates (pitted and chopped)
- 30 g celery (chopped or sliced
- 1-2 stalks parsley (chopped)
- 1 tablespoon capers
- 1 tablespoon extra-virgin olive oil
- 1 tablespoon lemon juice
- Salt& pepper

Method:

1. Drain and flake the tuna. Clean and chopped the vegetables.

2. Mix all the ingredients in a large salad bowl. Enjoy.

DINNER

Berry Juice. Use the same recipe as above.

(DAY 3)
BREAKFAST

Green Juice with Blueberries (1 serving)

(ALSO SUITABLE FOR MID-MORNING SNACK OR AFTERNOON TEA)

Ingredients:

- 1 cup blueberries
- 1 green apple (cored and cut)
- 50 g celery
- 75 g kale
- cucumber (peeled and cut)

Method:

1. Clean the vegetables and fruits. Juice or blend the fruits and vegetables.
2. Use a fine mesh strainer to strain the juice if you like. This is optional.
3. You may add some water to dilute the juice before drinking.

LUNCH

Tofu-Veggie Stir-Fry (1-2 servings)

Ingredients:

1. 14-0unce package firm or extra-firm tofu (can replace tofu with lean Chicken/turkey)
2. 1 cup kale
3. 1 cup rocket or arugula
4. 1 small red onion (peeled and chopped)
5. 1 clove garlic (minced)
6. A small handful walnuts (chopped)
7. stalk parsley (chopped)
8. 1 tablespoon extra-virgin olive oil
9. 1-2 bird's eye chilli (optional)
10. 50 g buckwheat or buckwheat noodle (prepared according to the packet instructions
11. Seasoning5: salt, pepper, sesame oil, soy sauce or tamari sauce, oyster sauce, chilli sauce, etc.

Method:

1. Pre-heat the oven to 400 "F.

2. Take half of the tofu and place between two clean towels or several layers of paper towels to dry the tofu.

3. When it is dry, roughly cut it into 1inch cubes.

4. Arrange the tofu on parchment-lined baking sheet and bake for 25- 35 minutes. Flip them once halfway through the baking. Baking the tofu will dry it up and produce a moat-like texture. If you prefer an even firmer texture, continue baking for another 10 minutes or more. Just don't burn the tofu. If you are using

lean chicken or turkey instead of tofu, skip step 1-4. Stir fry the chicken in the wok or pan.

5. Heat a large wok or frying pan. Add the kale with some water. Cook it for a few minutes until it wilts. Take It out and cool under running water to keep the colour.

6. Dry the pan and heat up the oil in the pan. Add the garlic and onion. Fry them for about 2 minutes.

7. Add the tofu into the pan. Add some water, about 1/3 cup to produce some gravy. Add your preferred seasonings such as soy sauce, oyster sauce and chili sauce

8. Add in the kale and arugula. Simmer for about 1 - 2 minutes.

9. Dish out and garnish with the chopped walnuts and parsley.

10. Serve with the prepared buckwheat.

DINNER

Green Juice with Blueberries. Follow the recipe above.

(DAY 4)

BREAKFAST

Sweet Green Juice (1 serving)

(ALSO SUITABLE FOR MID-MORNING SNACK OR
AFTERNOON TEA)

Ingredients

- 50 g kale or 1 cup packed
- 30 g celery
- green apple
- 1 handful blueberries
- ½ cucumber (peeled and cut)
- ½ teaspoon matcha green tea

Method:

1. Juice or blend all the ingredients except the green tea. Add the green tea at the end and blitz for a few seconds.
2. Use a fine mesh strainer to strain the juice before drinking (optional). Top-up with water if needed.

LUNCH

Teriyaki Salmon (2 servings)

Ingredients:

- 2 salmon filets (medium size)
- 1 clove garlic (minced
- 1/8 teaspoon grated ginger root
- 2 small red onions (chopped)
- 2 tablespoons light soy sauce
- 1 ½ tablespoon maple syrup/agave/natural honey
- 1 tablespoon mixing /rice wine
- 1 ½ tablespoons extra-virgin olive oil
- 2 stalks chopped parsley (for garnishing)
- Salt and pepper

Method:

1. Prepare the dressing by mixing the garlic, grated ginger, onion, soy sauce, maple syrup, mixing and halt tablespoon olive oil in a bowl.
2. Season the salmon fillets with salt and pepper. Pour the prepared dressing over the salmons and coat evenly: Cover and keep in the refrigerator to marinate for at least 1 hour,

3. Heat one tablespoon of the olive oil in a non-stick pan. Add the salmon, skin side down and cook for about 2 minutes.

4. Pour the marinade over the salmon. Add some water to the pan and baste the salmons with the sauce. Cook for about 2 minutes until the salmons turn opaque halfway up the sides.

5. Turn the salmons over to cook the other side for 3 4 minutes. Keep basting with the sauce. Add more water if the sauce is too thick. Adjust the seasoning if necessary.

6. Dish out the salmons. Garnish with the chopped parsley. Enjoy 1 fillet far lunch and reserve the other for dinner.

7. Serve the salmon with cooked buckwheat or an Apple Walnut Salad.

Apple Walnut Salad (1-2 servings)

Ingredients:

- 1 green apple (cored and diced/sliced)
- 1 small red onion (diced)
- 50 g celery (diced or sliced thinly)
- 50 g rocket/arugula (or 1 cup packed)
- 1 tomato (diced or sliced)
- ¼ cup walnuts (chopped)
- ½ cup medjool dates (pitted and chopped)
- 1 teaspoon maple syrup/agave/natural honey
- 1 tablespoon lemon juice
- 1 tablespoons reduced-calorie mayonnaise/non-fat sour cream
- 1 stalk chopped parsley (for garnishing)
- Salt and pepper

Method:

1. Mix the apples with the lemon juice in a bowl.
2. Add the celery, walnuts, tomato, onion, dates and rocket. Mix the mayonnaise with the syrup and fold into the salad mixture.
3. Season with salt and pepper. Garnish with the chopped parsley.

DINNER

Teriyaki Salmon

Enjoy the second portion of the salmon. Serve with Apple Walnut Salad

cooked buckwheat or other simple salad.

(DAY 5)

BREAKFAST

Pita Pizza (1 serving)

Ingredients

- 1 pita whole-meal pita bread (6 inch-diameter)
- 1 tomato (diced)
- 1 small red onion (chopped)
- 50 g rocket/arugula or 1 cup packed
- 1 stalk parsley/lavage (chopped)
- 1 tablespoon capers
- 1 tablespoon grated parmesan chees
- ¼ cup feta cheese/shredded mozzarella cheese
- Salt and pepper

Method

1. Heat ne oven to broil and arrange a rack In the middle.

2. Place the pita on a broiler pan and sprinkle with the feta/mozzarella cheese. Arrange the rocket over the cheese. Leave a small space in the center of the pita.

3. Crack an egg into the center of the pita. Sprinkle over with the red onion, tomato, caper, olive oil, salt and pepper.

4. Broil the pita until the egg white has set, about 6- 7 minutes (your preference).

5. Remove the pan iron the oven and transfer the pita to a plate. Sprinkle with the parmesan cheese and garnish with the parsley/lavage.

LUNCH

Refreshing Green Juice (1 serving)

(ALSO SUITABLE FOR MID-MORNING SNACK OR AFTERNOON TEA)

Ingredients:

- 50 g kale or rocket (or 1 cup packed)
- 1 green apple (cut and cared)
- 150 g celery
- ½ lemon
- ½ teaspoon matcha green tea
- ½ cucumber (peeled and cut)

Method:

1. Blend or blitz all the ingredients except the lemon and green tea. Squeeze the lemon into the mixture and add the green tea. Blitz for a few seconds.

2. Use a fine mesh strainer to strain the juice before drinking (optional). Top up with water if desired.

DINNER

Meat Loaf Pita Sandwich (1 servings)

Ingredients

- 1 meat loaf (from Day 1)
- 1 whole meal pita bread (6 inch-diameter)
- 1 tomato (diced)
- 1 small red onion (chopped)
- 1 stalk parsley/lavage (chopped)
- 50 g rocket/arugula (or 1 cup packed)
- 1 tablespoon lemon juice
- 1 tablespoon extra-virgin olive oil
- ¼ crumbled feta cheese (optional)
- Salt and pepper

Method:

1. Reheat the meat loaf in the microwave. Slice or crumble the meat loaf and divide into two portions

2. Mix the tomato, onion, parsley/lavage, rocket, olive oil, lemon juice, salt and pepper. Stir In the feta cheese.

3. Cut the pita bread in half. Stuff each half with a mixture of meat loaf and the salad above. Enjoy.

(DAY 6)

BREAKFAST

Soy Berry Smoothie (1 serving)

(ALSO SUITABLE FOR MID-MORNING SNACK OR AFTERNOON TEA)

Ingredients:

1 cup fresh strawberries/blueberries (or frozen)

1 cup unsweetened vanilla soymilk

Method:

1. Blend or blitz all the ingredients. Enjoy.

OR

Berry Yoghurt (1 serving)
Ingredients:

½ cup vanilla fat-free yoghurt

½ cup strawberries/blueberries

Method:

1. Mix all the ingredients. Enjoy.

LUNCH

Lentil Curry (2 servings)

Ingredients:

50 g rod or yellow lentils

1 large potato or sweet potato (peeled and cubed)

1 clove garlic (minced)

1 medium red onion or 3 small red onions (chopped) tomato (quartered) tablespoons turmeric

1 tablespoon curry paste/powder

2 cups vegetable/chicken broth

½ cup low fat milk

½ cup plain yoghurt (non-fat)

1 teaspoon cooking oil

2 stalks parsley (for garnishing)

Salt and pepper

Method:

1. Prepare the lentils the day before (on Day 2). Place the lentils in a sieve or colander and rinse under running tap water. Put the lentils inside a bowl/container and add enough tap water to cover the top.

Cover the bowl/container and refrigerate. Leave it to soak overnight. This will soften and shorten the cooking time. It is not a problem if you skip this stop. The cooking time will be slightly longer.

2. Heat the oil in a pot and add the garlic and onion. Fry for about 2-3 minutes.

3. Drain the lentils and add it to the pot. Add the tomato, potato, turmeric and curry spices. Fry for about 2 minutes.

 4. Pour in the vegetable broth and milk. Add same seasonings

5. Bring the mixture to a boil, then reduce to a simmer. Simmer the mixture for 20-30 minutes or until the lentils and potatoos have soften.

6. Add more liquid if you want it more 'soupy.' Also add the yoghurt. Add more seasonings if necessary.

7. Divide the curry into 2 portions. Enjoy one portion for lunch and the next for dinner

8. Serve the curry with cooked buckwheat if you like.

Suggestions:

1. You can add other types of vegetables like pumpkin, squash, cauliflower, carrots, peas, etc.

2. You can also add chopped dried apricots or raisins to make it sweeter.

3. Instead of lentils, use only vegetables to make a vegetable curry

DINNER

Lentil Curry

Enjoy the second portion of the lentil curry. Serve with cooked buckwheat or a salad.

(DAY 7)

BREAKFAST

Sweet Green Juice (1 serving)

(ALSO SUITABLE FOR MID-MORNING SNACK OR AFTERNOON TEA)

Ingredients

- 50 g kale or 1 cup packed
- 30 g celery
- green apple
- 1 handful blueberries
- ½ cucumber (peeled and cut)
- ½ teaspoon matcha green tea

Method:

8. Juice or blend all the ingredients except the green tea. Add the green tea at the end and blitz for a few seconds.
9. Use a fine mesh strainer to strain the juice before drinking (optional). Topup with water if needed.

LUNCH

Teriyaki Salmon (2 servings)

Ingredients:

- 2 salmon filets (medium size)
- 1 clove garlic (minced
- 1/8 teaspoon grated ginger root
- 2 small red onions (chopped)
- 2 tablespoons light soy sauce
- 1 ½ tablespoon maple syrup/agave/natural honey
- 1 tablespoon mixing /rice wine
- 1 ½ tablespoons extra-virgin olive oil
- 2 stalks chopped parsley (for garnishing)
- Salt and pepper

Method:

3. Prepare the dressing by mixing the garlic, grated ginger, onion, soy sauce, maple syrup, mixing and halt tablespoon olive oil In a bowl.
4. Season the salmon fillets with salt and pepper. Pour the prepared dressing over the salmons and coat evenly: Cover and keep in the refrigerator to marinate for at least 1 hour,

10. Heat one tablespoon of the olive oil in a non-stick pan. Add the salmon, skin side down and cook for about 2 minutes.

11. Pour the marinade over the salmon. Add some water to the pan and baste the salmons with the sauce. Cook for about 2 minutes until the salmons turn opaque halfway up the sides.

12. Turn the salmons over to cook the other side for 3 4 minutes. Keep basting with the sauce. Add more water if the sauce is too thick. Adjust the seasoning if necessary.

13. Dish out the salmons. Garnish with the chopped parsley. Enjoy 1 fillet far lunch and reserve the other for dinner.

14. Serve the salmon with cooked buckwheat or an Apple Walnut Salad.

Apple Walnut Salad (1-2 servings)

Ingredients:

- 1 green apple (cored and diced/sliced)
- 1 small red onion (diced)
- 50 g celery (diced or sliced thinly)
- 50 g rocket/arugula (or 1 cup packed)
- 1 tomato (diced or sliced)
- ¼ cup walnuts (chopped)
- ½ cup medjool dates (pitted and chopped)

- 1 teaspoon maple syrup/agave/natural honey
- 1 tablespoon lemon juice
- 1 tablespoons reduced-calorie mayonnaise/non-fat sour cream
- 1 stalk chopped parsley (for garnishing)
- Salt and pepper

Method:

4. Mix the apples with the lemon juice in a bowl.
5. Add the celery, walnuts, tomato, onion, dates and rocket. Mix the mayonnaise with the syrup and fold into the salad mixture.
6. Season with salt and pepper. Garnish with the chopped parsley.

DINNER

Teriyaki Salmon

Enjoy the second portion of the salmon. Serve with Apple Walnut Salad

cooked buckwheat or other simple salad.

CHAPTER 8:
MAINTAINING

It is recommended that you repeat the diet phases as desired until you reach your weight loss goal.

You should drink a glass of green juice daily to maintain the sirtuin effect.

I believe that the sirt diet is a lifestyle change rather than a single diet.

Before trying the Sirt Food Diet, you should probably consider the extreme difficulties that even dietitians have noticed. Because it limits carbohydrates, it mainly focuses on short-term weight loss. So if you want to maintain weight loss, another diet or diet may be easier to manage in the long run.

Rick Hay comments: "The Sirt diet is very restrictive and less balanced than the Keto or Paleo diet. It focuses on calorie counting and requires you to cut out the main food groups. You also need to reduce your portions, especially the first week Another disadvantage is the fact that the diet lacks important nutrients such as calcium and iron.

"If you are not used to restricting your daily food intake, you may experience nausea, dizziness, difficulty concentrating, tiredness and headache."

If the food looks healthy enough and you can practically do without the sirt food diet, is this a good choice?

Experts: "In terms of nutrient density, foods with a high sirthrin content also offer a good nutrient content that is generally associated with an improvement in health," says Lola. "In addition to reducing calories, this leads to results," says Lola.

"It may be that considering the foods that are normally off-limits in diets is actually the plan's secret of success," says Sophie. "If you feel like you are eating foods like chocolate and red wine, you will probably feel less constrained than cutting them off your diet."

"Maintaining this in the long term can be very difficult and often requires major changes," she adds. Life changes and limitations, which may not all be positive. The effects on our mood of gaining weight after a diet have also been identified as the main drivers for the return to comfortable eating and less healthy eating habits. ""

"We will certainly not recommend the sirt food diet in my clinics or as a medical treatment for weight loss," says Sophie. "Although we can promote certain healthy foods, strict regulations and the replacement of meals with juices often cause difficulties in people's eating relationships and can cause us to lose sight of how excessive weight loss is."

CHAPTER 9:
SHOPPING LIST

Ingredients that you should always have at home for the Sirtfood Diet

You should always have the following ingredients at home when you follow the goggins and mats diet. So this is your ultimate shopping list!

Vegetables, fresh

These vegetables occur almost every day. So always keep it in stock.

- Kale
- garlic
- Thai chili (Bird's eye chili)
- Red onions
- beverages
- Black coffee)
- Red wine (Pinot Noir, aka Pinot Noir)
- Tea (green, black, white)
- water

- Herbs, fresh

These herbs are used so often that you should always have them fresh at home. It is best to pull them yourself!

Leaf parsley

- Ginger (even if it's not an herb, let's put it in here ...)
- Lovage
- Herbs and spices, dried
- Curry mix; mild, medium or hot to taste
- coriander
- Cumin (cumin)
- turmeric
- sage
- Mustard seeds
- Tamari or Soyausce
- nuts
- Walnuts
- Fruit, fresh
- Lemons
- Oils

- Extra virgin olive oil
- Other foods
- Buckwheat
- Chocolate (at least 85% cocoa)
- Soba noodles

THE TOP SIRTFOODS

- Buckwheat
- Capers
- Celery
- Chili
- Chocolate
- Coffee
- Extra Virgin Olive Oil
- Green Tea – ideally matcha
- Kale
- Lovage
- Medjool Dates
- Parsley
- Red Chicory
- Red Onion

- Red Wine
- Rocket
- Soy
- Strawberries
- Turmeric
- Walnuts

Chapter 10:

Recipes

An apple and an egg

Ingredients:

- 2 pieces Egg
- 1 piece Apple (in cubes)
- ½ pieces Onion (finely chopped.)
- ½ pieces Cucumber (in cubes)
- 200 g Corn salad

Preparation:

1. Boil the eggs hard for 8 minutes, scare them under cold water and peel them.
2. Mix the lettuce, cucumber, onion and apple in a large bowl.
3. Cut the egg into cubes and put them in the bowl.
4. Drizzle the salad with olive oil and season with salt and pepper.

Sweet potato salad with bacon

Ingredients:

- 5 slices Bacon
- 2 pieces Sweet potato (peeled and diced)
- 3 cloves Garlic (pressed)
- 4 tablespoon Lime juice
- 3 tablespoon Olive oil
- 1 tablespoon Balsamic vinegar

Preparation:

1. Preheat the oven to 220 ° C and cover a baking sheet with parchment paper.
2. Place the bacon on the baking sheet and bake until crispy in the oven (approx. 20 minutes).
3. Take the bacon off the baking sheet, let it cool and chop it.
4. Mix the sweet potato cubes with garlic on the same baking sheet, drizzle with a little mild olive oil and fry them in the oven for about 30 minutes.
5. Prepare a dressing made from olive oil, vinegar, and lime juice by mixing them in a bowl.
6. Take the potato cubes out of the oven, mix them with the bacon pieces and drizzle them with the dressing.
7. If you like, add rocket and/or pine nuts at the end.

Salad with melon and ham

Ingredients:

- 1 piece Cantaloupe melon
- 8 slices Serrano ham chopped
- 200 g Rocket
- 1 piece Cucumber (sliced)
- 1 piece Red onion (rings)
- 3 tablespoon Olive oil

Preparation:

1. Quarter the melon. Remove the seeds with a spoon, cut the peel and cut the melon into equal parts.
2. Wrap melon parts in ham.
3. Mix the arugula with the cucumber and onion in a bowl.
4. Drizzle the salad with olive oil.
5. Spread this on the plates and place the wrapped melon parts on it.

Paleo Chicken Wraps

Ingredients:

- 2 pieces Egg
- 240 ml Almond milk
- 1 tcaspoon Olive oil (mild)
- $1/4$ TL Celtic sea salt
- 75 g Tapioca flour
- Coconut flour3 tablespoon
- Chicken breast10 slices
- mixed salad2 hands

Preparation:

1. Whisk the eggs in a bowl, then add almond milk, olive oil, and salt.
2. Add tapioca and coconut flour and stir with a whisk until you get an even batter.
3. Grease a pan and pour 1/6 of the batter into the pan.
4. The wraps should have a diameter of approx. 15 cm.
5. Fry the wraps on both sides until golden brown.
6. Repeat this step with the rest of the dough.
7. Fill the wraps with chicken and possibly additional salad or raw vegetables as you like.

Chocolate Breakfast Muffins

Ingredients:

- 250 g Almond paste
- 3 pieces Banana (ripe)
- 2 pieces Egg
- 1 teaspoon Vanilla extract
- $^1/_2$ teaspoon Tartar baking powder
- 100 g Chocolate chips

Preparation:

1. Preheat the oven to 200 ° C and prepare a baking sheet with paper or silicone muffin tins.
2. Place all ingredients (except the optional chocolate chips) in a food processor and mix them into a smooth, sticky dough.
3. Optional: add pieces of chocolate and stir
4. Optional: add pieces of chocolate and stir
5. Place the dough in the muffin tins and bake until golden brown and cooked in about 12-15 minutes.

Apple Cinnamon Wraps

Ingredient:

For the wraps:

- 2 pieces Egg (beaten)
- 240 ml Almond milk
- 1 teaspoon Olive oil (mild)
- $^1/_4$ TL Celtic sea salt
- 75 g Tapioca flour
- 3 tablespoons Coconut flour

For garnish:

- 1 tablespoon Ghee
- 1 piece Apple
- 1 teaspoon Cinnamon
- 1 hand Cranberries
- 1 teaspoon Lemon juice

Preparation:

1. Whisk the eggs in a bowl, then add almond milk, olive oil, and salt.
2. Add the tapioca and coconut flour and stir with a whisk until you get an even batter.
3. Grease a pan and pour 1/6 of the batter into the pan.
4. The wraps should have a diameter of approx. 15 cm.
5. Fry the wraps on both sides until golden brown.
6. Heat the ghee in a pan.
7. Add the diced apple, cinnamon, cranberries and lemon juice and cook over medium heat until the apple is soft.
8. Spoon the apple onto the wrap and fold it into a roll.
9. Enjoy it!

Avocado and salmon salad buffet

Ingredients:

- $^1/_2$ pieces Cucumber
- 1 piece Avocado
- $^1/_2$ pieces Red onion
- 250 g mixed salad
- 4 slices smoked salmon

Preparation:

1. Cut the cucumber and avocado into cubes and chop the onion.
2. Spread the lettuce leaves on deep plates and spread the cucumber, avocado, and onion over the lettuce.
3. Season with salt and pepper (you can also add a little olive oil to the salad).
4. Place smoked salmon slices on top and serve.

Paleo-force bars

Ingredients:

- 10 pieces Medjoul dates (cored)
- 100 g Grated coconut
- 100 g crushed linseed
- 75 g Cashew nuts
- 60 g Coconut oil

Preparation:

1. Place all ingredients in a food processor and pulse until a sticky and granular dough is formed.
2. Line a small baking sheet with parchment paper.
3. Spread the mixture on the bottom of the baking sheet and press down firmly.
4. Let them solidify and harden them in the freezer for a few hours.
5. After the mixture has hardened, cut it into bars.
6. If you want to pack them as individual snacks, wrap the bars in cling film or baking paper.

Vinaigrette

Ingredients:

- 4 teaspoons Mustard yellow
- 4 tablespoon White wine vinegar
- 1 teaspoon Honey
- 165 ml Olive oil

Preparation:

1. Whisk the mustard, vinegar, and honey in a bowl with a whisk until they are well mixed.
2. Add the olive oil in small amounts while whisking with a whisk until the vinaigrette is thick.
3. Season with salt and pepper.

Spicy Ras-el-Hanout dressing

Ingredients:

- 125 ml Olive oil
- 1 piece Lemon (the juice)
- 2 teaspoons Honey
- 1 ½ teaspoons Ras el Hanout
- ½ pieces Red pepper

Preparation:

1. Remove the seeds from the chili pepper.
2. Chop the chili pepper as finely as possible.
3. Place the pepper in a bowl with lemon juice, honey, and Ras-El-Hanout and whisk with a whisk.
4. Then add the olive oil drop by drop while continuing to whisk.

Chicken rolls with pesto

Ingredients:

- 2 tablespoon Pine nuts
- 25 g Yeast flakes
- 1 clove Garlic (chopped)
- 15 g fresh basil
- 85 ml Olive oil
- 2 pieces Chicken breast

Preparation:

1. Preheat the oven to 175 ° C.
2. Roast the pine nuts in a dry pan over medium heat for 3 minutes until golden brown. Place on a plate and set aside.
3. Put the pine nuts, yeast flakes and garlic in a food processor and grind them finely.
4. Add the basil and oil and mix briefly until you get a pesto.
5. Season with salt and pepper.
6. Place each piece of chicken breast between 2 pieces of cling film
7. Beat with a saucepan or rolling pin until the chicken breast is about 0.6 cm thick.
8. Remove the cling film and spread the pesto on the chicken.
9. Roll up the chicken breasts and use cocktail skewers to hold them together.
10. Season with salt and pepper.
11. Melt the coconut oil in a pan and brown the chicken rolls on all sides over high heat.
12. Put the chicken rolls in a baking dish, place in the oven and bake for 15-20 minutes until they are done.
13. Slice the rolls diagonally and serve with the rest of the pesto.
14. Goes well with a tomato salad.

Mustard

Ingredients:

- 60 g Mustard seeds
- 60 ml Water
- 60 ml Apple cider vinegar
- 2 teaspoons Lemon juice
- 90 g Honey
- ½ teaspoon dried turmeric

Preparation:

1. Put mustard seeds, water and vinegar in a glass, close well and leave in the fridge for 12 hours.
2. Put all ingredients in a tall measuring cup the next day.
3. Use your hand blender to puree everything.
4. Try the mustard and add some honey or salt.
5. Store the mustard in a clean glass in the fridge, it will keep for at least 3 weeks.

Vegetarian curry from the crock pot:

Ingredients:

- 4 pieces Carrot
- 2 pieces Sweet potato
- 1 piece Onion
- 3 cloves Garlic
- 2 tablespoon Curry powder
- 1 teaspoon Ground caraway (ground)
- ¼ teaspoon Chili powder
- ¼ TL Celtic sea salt
- 1 pinch Cinnamon
- 100 ml Vegetable broth
- 400 g Tomato cubes (can)
- 250 g Sweet peas
- 2 tablespoon Tapioca flour

Preparation:

1. Roughly chop vegetables and potatoes and press garlic. Halve the sugar snap peas.
2. Put the carrots, sweet potatoes and onions in the slow cooker.
3. Mix tapioca flour with curry powder, cumin, chili powder, salt and cinnamon and sprinkle this mixture on the vegetables.
4. Pour the vegetable broth over it.
5. Close the lid of the slow cooker and let it simmer for 6 hours on a low setting.
6. Stir in the tomatoes and sugar snap peas for the last hour.
7. Cauliflower rice is a great addition to this dish.

Fried cauliflower rice:

Ingredients:

- 1 piece Cauliflower
- 2 tablespoon Coconut oil
- 1 piece Red onion
- 4 cloves Garlic
- 60 ml Vegetable broth
- 1.5 cm fresh ginger
- 1 teaspoon Chili flakes
- ½ pieces Carrot
- ½ pieces Red bell pepper
- ½ pieces Lemon (the juice)
- 2 tablespoon Pumpkin seeds
- 2 tablespoon fresh coriander

Preparation:

1. Cut the cauliflower into small rice grains in a food processor.
2. Finely chop the onion, garlic and ginger, cut the carrot into thin strips, dice the bell pepper and finely chop the herbs.
3. Melt 1 tablespoon of coconut oil in a pan and add half of the onion and garlic to the pan and fry briefly until translucent.
4. Add cauliflower rice and season with salt.

5. Pour in the broth and stir everything until it evaporates and the cauliflower rice is tender.
6. Take the rice out of the pan and set it aside.
7. Melt the rest of the coconut oil in the pan and add the remaining onions, garlic, ginger, carrots and peppers.
8. Fry for a few minutes until the vegetables are tender. Season them with a little salt.
9. Add the cauliflower rice again, heat the whole dish and add the lemon juice.
10. Garnish with pumpkin seeds and coriander before serving.

Mediterranean paleo pizza:

Ingredients:

For the pizza crusts:

- 120 g Tapioca flour
- 1 teaspoon Celtic sea salt
- 2 tablespoon Italian spice mix
- 45 g Coconut flour
- 120 ml Olive oil (mild)
- Water (warm) 120 ml
- Egg (beaten) 1 piece

For covering:

- 2 tablespoon Tomato paste (can)
- ½ pieces Zucchini
- ½ pieces Eggplant
- 2 pieces Tomato
- 2 tablespoon Olive oil (mild)
- 1 tablespoon Balsamic vinegar

Preparation:

1. Preheat the oven to 190 ° C and line a baking sheet with parchment paper.
2. Cut the vegetables into thin slices.
3. Mix the tapioca flour with salt, Italian herbs and coconut flour in a large bowl.
4. Pour in olive oil and warm water and stir well.

5. Then add the egg and stir until you get an even dough.
6. If the dough is too thin, add 1 tablespoon of coconut flour at a time until it is the desired thickness. Always wait a few minutes before adding more coconut flour, as it will take some time to absorb the moisture. The intent is to get a soft, sticky dough.
7. Divide the dough into two parts and spread them in flat circles on the baking sheet (or make 1 large sheet of pizza as shown in the picture).
8. Bake in the oven for about 10 minutes.
9. Brush the pizza with tomato paste and spread the aubergines, zucchini and tomato overlapping on the pizza.
10. Drizzle the pizza with olive oil and bake in the oven for another 10-15 minutes.
11. Drizzle balsamic vinegar over the pizza before serving.

d chicken and broccolini :

Ingredients:

- 2 tablespoon Coconut oil
- 400 g Chicken breast
- Bacon cubes 150 g
- Broccolini 250 g

Preparation:

1. Cut the chicken into cubes.
2. Melt the coconut oil in a pan over medium heat and brown the chicken with the bacon cubes and cook through.
3. Season with chili flakes, salt and pepper.
4. Add broccolini and fry.
5. Stack on a plate and enjoy!

Braised leek with pine nuts:

Ingredients:

- 20 g Ghee
- 2 teaspoon Olive oil
- 2 pieces Leek
- 150 ml Vegetable broth
- fresh parsley
- 1 tablespoon fresh oregano
- 1 tablespoon Pine nuts (roasted)

Preparation:

1. Cut the leek into thin rings and finely chop the herbs. Roast the pine nuts in a dry pan over medium heat.
2. Melt the ghee together with the olive oil in a large pan.
3. Cook the leek until golden brown for 5 minutes, stirring constantly.
4. Add the vegetable broth and cook for another 10 minutes until the leek is tender.
5. Stir in the herbs and sprinkle the pine nuts on the dish just before serving.

Sweet and sour pan with cashew nuts:

Ingredients:

- 2 tablespoon Coconut oil
- 2 pieces Red onion
- 2 pieces yellow bell pepper
- 250 g White cabbage
- 150 g Pak choi
- 50 g Mung bean sprouts
- 4 pieces Pineapple slices
- 50 g Cashew nuts

For the sweet and sour sauce:

- 60 ml Apple cider vinegar
- 4 tablespoon Coconut blossom sugar
- 1½ tablespoon Tomato paste
- 1 teaspoon Coconut-Aminos
- 2 teaspoon Arrowroot powder
- 75 ml Water

Preparation:

1. Roughly cut the vegetables.
2. Mix the arrow root with five tablespoons of cold water into a paste.
3. Then put all the other ingredients for the sauce in a saucepan and add the arrowroot paste for binding.
4. Melt the coconut oil in a pan and fry the onion.
5. Add the bell pepper, cabbage, pak choi and bean sprouts and stir-fry until the vegetables become a little softer.
6. Add the pineapple and cashew nuts and stir a few more times.
7. Pour a little sauce over the wok dish and serve.

Casserole with spinach and eggplant

Ingredients:

- 1 piece Eggplant
- 2 pieces Onion
- Olive oil 3 tablespoon
- Spinach (fresh) 450 g
- Tomatoes 4 pieces
- Egg 2 pieces
- 60 ml Almond milk
- 2 teaspoons Lemon juice
- 4 tablespoon Almond flour

Preparation:

1. Preheat the oven to 200 ° C.
2. Cut the eggplants, onions and tomatoes into slices and sprinkle salt on the eggplant slices.
3. Brush the eggplants and onions with olive oil and fry them in a grill pan.
4. Shrink the spinach in a large saucepan over moderate heat and drain in a sieve.
5. Put the vegetables in layers in a greased baking dish: first the eggplant, then the spinach and then the onion and the tomato. Repeat this again.
6. Whisk eggs with almond milk, lemon juice, salt and pepper and pour over the vegetables.
7. Sprinkle almond flour over the dish and bake in the oven for about 30 to 40 minutes.

Vegetarian paleo ratatouille:

Ingredients:

- 200 g Tomato cubes (can)
- $^1/_2$ pieces Onion
- 2 cloves Garlic
- $^1/_4$ teaspoon dried oregano
- $^1/_4$ TL Chili flakes
- 2 tablespoon Olive oil
- 1 piece Eggplant
- 1 piece Zucchini
- 1 piece hot peppers
- 1 teaspoon dried thyme

Preparation:

1. Preheat the oven to 180 ° C and lightly grease a round or oval shape.
2. Finely chop the onion and garlic.
3. Mix the tomato cubes with garlic, onion, oregano and chilli flakes, season with salt and pepper and put on the bottom of the baking dish.
4. Use a mandolin, a cheese slicer or a sharp knife to cut the eggplant, zucchini and hot pepper into very thin slices.
5. Put the vegetables in a bowl (make circles, start at the edge and work inside).
6. Drizzle the remaining olive oil on the vegetables and sprinkle with thyme, salt and pepper.
7. Cover the baking dish with a piece of parchment paper and bake in the oven for 45 to 55 minutes.
8. Enjoy it!

Courgette and broccoli soup:

Ingredient:

- 2 tablespoon Coconut oil
- 1 piece Red onion
- 2 cloves Garlic
- 300 g Broccoli
- 1 piece Zucchini
- 750 ml Vegetable broth

Preparation:

1. Finely chop the onion and garlic, cut the broccoli into florets and the zucchini into slices.
2. Melt the coconut oil in a soup pot and fry the onion with the garlic.
3. Cook the zucchini for a few minutes.
4. Add broccoli and vegetable broth and simmer for about 5 minutes.
5. Puree the soup with a hand blender and season with salt and pepper.

Frittata with spring onions and asparagus:

(scallions)

Ingredients:

- 5 pieces Egg
- 80 ml Almond milk
- 2 tablespoon Coconut oil
- 1 clove Garlic
- 100 g Asparagus tips
- 4 pieces Spring onions
- 1 teaspoon Tarragon
- 1 pinch Chilli flakes

Preparation:

1. Preheat the oven to 220 ° C.
2. Squeeze the garlic and finely chop the spring onions.
3. Whisk the eggs with the almond milk and season with salt and pepper.
4. Melt 1 tablespoon of coconut oil in a medium-sized cast iron pan and briefly fry the onion and garlic with the asparagus.
5. Remove the vegetables from the pan and melt the remaining coconut oil in the pan.
6. Pour in the egg mixture and half of the entire vegetable.
7. Place the pan in the oven for 15 minutes until the egg has solidified.
8. Then take the pan out of the oven and pour the rest of the egg with the vegetables into the pan.
9. Place the pan in the oven again for 15 minutes until the egg is nice and loose.
10. Sprinkle the tarragon and chilli flakes on the dish before serving.

Cucumber salad with lime and coriander (Cilantro)

Ingredients:

- 1 piece Red onion
- 2 pieces Cucumber
- 2 pieces Lime (juice)
- 2 tablespoon fresh coriander

Preparation:

1. Cut the onion into rings and thinly slice the cucumber. Chop the coriander finely.
2. Place the onion rings in a bowl and season with about half a tablespoon of salt.
3. Rub it in well and then fill the bowl with water.
4. Pour off the water and then rinse the onion rings thoroughly (in a sieve).
5. Put the cucumber slices together with onion, lime juice, coriander and olive oil in a salad bowl and stir everything well.
6. Season with a little salt.
7. You can keep this dish in the refrigerator in a covered bowl for a few days.

bell pepper filled with egg:

gredients:

- 1 tablespoon Coconut oil
- 4 pieces Egg
- 1 piece Tomato
- 1 pinch Chilli flakes
- ¼ teaspoon Ground cumin
- ¼ teaspoon Paprika powder
- ½ pieces Avocado
- 1 piece green peppers
- 2 tablespoon fresh coriander

Preparation:

1. Cut the tomatoes and avocado into cubes and finely chop the fresh coriander.
2. Melt the coconut oil in a pan over medium heat, beat the eggs in the pan and add the tomato cubes.
3. Keep stirring until the eggs solidify and season with chilli, caraway, paprika, pepper, and salt.
4. Finally add the avocado.
5. Place the egg mixture in the pepper halves and garnish with fresh coriander.

Honey mustard dressing

Ingredients:

- 4 tablespoon Olive oil
- $1^1/_2$ teaspoon Honey
- $1^1/_2$ teaspoon Mustard
- 1 teaspoon Lemon juice
- 1 pinch Salt

Preparation:

1. Mix olive oil, honey, mustard and lemon juice into an even dressing with a whisk.
2. Season with salt.

Paleo chocolate wraps with fruits

Ingredients:

- 4 pieces Egg
- 100 ml Almond milk
- 2 tablespoons Arrowroot powder
- 4 tablespoons Chestnut flour
- 1 tablespoon Olive oil (mild)
- 2 tablespoons Maple syrup
- 2 tablespoons Cocoa powder
- 1 tablespoon Coconut oil
- 1 piece Banana
- 2 pieces Kiwi (green)
- 2 pieces Mandarins

Preparation:

1. Mix all ingredients (except fruit and coconut oil) into an even dough.
2. Melt some coconut oil in a small pan and pour a quarter of the batter into it.
3. Bake it like a pancake baked on both sides.
4. Place the fruit in a wrap and serve it lukewarm.
5. A wonderfully sweet start to the day!

Chocolate sauce

Ingredients:

- 75 g Cocoa powder
- 250 ml Coconut milk (can)
- 95 pieces Dates
- 3 tablespoon Coconut oil
- ½ teaspoon Vanilla extract
- 1 pinch Salt

Preparation:

1. Put the dates in a bowl, pour boiling water over them and let them stand for 10 minutes.
2. Drain the dates.
3. Heat the coconut milk and coconut oil in a pan.
4. Put all the ingredients in a blender and puree into an even sauce.
5. Add some hot water if you think the sauce is too thick. (Mix them again if you add water).

Hot sauce

Ingredients:

- 2 pieces Tomato
- 2 pieces Red peppers
- 10 cloves Garlic
- 2 pieces Red pepper
- 250 ml White wine vinegar
- 2 tablespoons Olive oil
- 1 tablespoon Honey
- 1 tablespoon Celtic sea salt

Preparation:

1. Singe the tomatoes and peppers over your gas burner. (or in the oven at 220 ° C if you don't have a gas burner)
2. Let cool down.
3. Cut the paprika into pieces and remove the stones.
4. Heat a pan and roast the garlic (without oil) for a few minutes. Let cool down.
5. Clean the peppers, remove the seeds if necessary.
6. Put the tomatoes, peppers, garlic and peppers in a blender. Add 125 ml of water and puree well.
7. Pour the mixture into a saucepan and add the oil, honey, salt, and vinegar. Bring the mixture to a boil. Turn the heat down as soon as it boils and let it simmer for 5 minutes.
8. Let cool and check if the sauce still needs salt.
9. Put the sauce in a glass and let it rest in the fridge for 2 days. Thereupon she will soon burst with taste.
10. Before use; take a bowl and put a fine sieve on it. Pour the sauce over the sieve and press as far as possible with the convex side of the spoon.
11. You can throw away the residues remaining in the sieve.

Paleo breakfast salad with egg

Ingredients:

- 1 teaspoon Ghee
- 2 pieces Egg
- 1 hand Spinach
- ½ pieces Red bell pepper
- ¼ pieces Onion
- 50 g Carrot
- 50 g Cucumber
- 1 piece Tomato
- ½ pieces Avocado

Ingredients:

1. Chop the onion, cut the bell pepper into strips, cut the cucumber and avocado into cubes, grate the carrot and cut the tomato into wedges.
2. Melt the ghee in a pan over medium heat and beat the eggs into the pan.
3. In the meantime, prepare the salad by putting all the remaining ingredients on a plate.
4. Remove the eggs from the pan when the egg yolk is still a little soft, this looks like a delicious dressing! (or if you prefer a well-fried egg, drizzle your salad with some olive oil as a dressing).
5. Season with salt and pepper.

Caesar dressing

Ingredients:

- 250 ml Olive oil
- 2 tablespoons Lemon juice
- 4 pieces Anchovy fillet
- 2 tablespoon Mustard yellow
- 1 clove Garlic
- $^1/_2$ teaspoon Salt
- ½ teaspoon Black pepper

Preparation:

1. Remove the peel from the garlic and chop it finely.
2. Put all ingredients in a blender and puree evenly.
3. This dressing can be kept in the fridge for about 3 days.

Basil dressing

Ingredients:

- fresh basil100 g
- Shallots1 piece
- Garlic1 clove
- Olive oil (mild)125 ml
- White wine vinegar2 tablespoon

Preparation:

1. Finely chop the shallot and garlic.
2. Put the shallot, garlic, basil, olive oil and vinegar in a blender.
3. Mix it into an even mix.
4. Season the dressing and season with salt and pepper.
5. Place the dressing in a clean glass and store in the refrigerator. It stays fresh and tasty for at least 3 days.

Strawberry sauce

Ingredients:

- 225 g Strawberries
- 3 tablespoons Coconut blossom sugar
- 4 tablespoons Honey
- 125 ml Water
- 2 teaspoon Arrowroot powder

Preparation:

1. Roughly chop strawberries.
2. Put the strawberries in a pan with coconut blossom sugar and honey. Place the pan on medium heat.
3. In the meantime, mix the arrow roots with a whisk in the water. Add this mixture to the strawberries.
4. Heat the strawberries until they start to bubble and start to thicken. (Not cook!)
5. Your strawberry sauce is ready after about 15 minutes.
6. Store the sauce in the fridge in a clean glass.

Fresh chicory salad:

Ingredients:

- 1 piece Orange
- 1 piece Tomato
- $1/4$ pieces Cucumber
- $1/4$ pieces Red onion

Preparation:

1. Cut off the hard stem of the chicory and remove the leaves.
2. Peel the orange and cut the pulp into wedges.
3. Cut the tomatoes and cucumbers into small pieces.
4. Cut the red onion into thin half rings.
5. Place the chicory boats on a plate, spread the orange wedges, tomato, cucumber and red onion over the boats.
6. Drizzle some olive oil and fresh lemon juice on the dish.

Grilled vegetables and tomatoes

Ingredients:

- 1 piece Zucchini
- 1 piece Eggplant
- 3 pieces Tomatoes
- 1 piece Cucumber

Ingredients dressing:

- 4 tablespoons Olive oil
- 110 ml Orange juice (fresh)
- 1 tablespoon Apple cider vinegar
- 1 hand fresh basil

Preparation:

1. Cut all of the vegetables into equally thick slices (about half a centimeter).
2. Heat the grill pan and fry the zucchini and eggplant.
3. Season with salt and pepper while the zucchini and eggplant are fried.
4. Remove the basil leaves from the branches.
5. Spread the vegetables alternately on a plate.
6. Add a leaf of basil every now and then.
7. Mix the ingredients for the dressing and serve the dressing separately on the side.

Steak salad

Ingredients:

- 2 pieces Beef steak
- 2 cloves Garlic
- 1 piece Red onion
- 2 pieces Egg
- 1 hand Cherry tomatoes
- 2 hands Lettuce
- 1 piece Avocado
- $^1/_2$ pieces Cucumber
- 1 pinch Season white Salt
- 1 pinch Black pepper

Preparation:

1. Place the steaks in a flat bowl.
2. Pour the olive oil over the steaks and press the garlic over it. Turn the steaks a few times so that they are covered with oil and garlic.
3. Cover the meat and let it marinate for at least 1 hour.
4. Boil eggs.
5. Heat a grill pan and fry the steaks medium.
6. Take the steaks out of the pan, wrap them in aluminum foil and let them rest for 5 to 10 minutes.
7. Spread the lettuce on the plates.
8. Cut the steaks into slices and place them in the middle of the salad.

9. Cut the eggs into wedges, the cucumber into half-moons, the red onion into thin half-rings, the cherry tomatoes into halves and the avocado into slices.
10. Spread this around the steaks.
11. Drizzle over the olive oil and white wine vinegar and season with a little salt and pepper.

Zucchini salad with lemon chicken

Ingredients:

- 1 piece Zucchini
- 1 piece yellow zucchini
- 1 hand Cherry tomatoes
- 2 pieces Chicken breast
- 1 piece Lemon
- 2 tablespoons Olive oil

Preparation:

1. Use a meat mallet or a heavy pan to make the chicken fillets as thin as possible.
2. Put the fillets in a bowl.
3. Squeeze the lemon over the chicken and add the olive oil. Cover it and let it marinate for at least 1 hour.
4. Heat a pan over medium-high heat and fry the chicken until cooked through and browned.
5. Season with salt and pepper.
6. Make zucchini from the zucchini and put in a bowl.
7. Quarter the tomatoes and stir in the zucchini.
8. Slice the chicken fillets diagonally and place them on the salad.
9. Drizzle the salad with a little olive oil and season with salt and pepper.

ʜ salad with orange dressing

Ingredients

- $^1/_2$ fruit Salad
- 1 piece yellow bell pepper
- 1 piece Red pepper
- 100 g Carrot (grated)
- 1 hand Almonds

Ingredients dressing:

- 4 tablespoon Olive oil
- 110 ml Orange juice (fresh)
- 1 tablespoon Apple cider vinegar

Preparation:

1. Clean the peppers and cut them into long thin strips.
2. Tear off the lettuce leaves and cut them into smaller pieces.
3. Mix the salad with the peppers and the carrots processed with the Julienne peeler in a bowl.
4. Roughly chop the almonds and sprinkle over the salad.
5. Mix all the ingredients for the dressing in a bowl.
6. Pour the dressing over the salad just before serving.

Tomato and avocado salad

Ingredients:

- 1 piece Tomato
- 1 hand Cherry tomatoes
- $^1/_2$ pieces Red onion
- 1 piece Avocado
- Taste fresh oregano
- 1 $^1/_2$ EL Olive oil
- 1 teaspoon White wine vinegar
- 1 pinch Celtic sea salt

Preparation:

1. Cut the tomato into thick slices.
2. Cut half of the cherry tomatoes into slices and the other half in half.
3. Cut the red onion into super thin half rings. (or use a mandolin for this)
4. Cut the avocado into 6 parts.
5. Spread the tomatoes on a plate, place the avocado on top and sprinkle the red onion over them.
6. Sprinkle fresh oregano on the salad as desired.
7. Drizzle olive oil and vinegar on the salad with a pinch of salt.

Arugula with fruits and nuts

Ingredients:

- 75 g Arugula
- 2 pieces Peach
- $^{1}/_{2}$ pieces Red onion
- 1 hand Blueberries
- Pecans 1 hand

Ingredients dressing:

- $^{1}/_{2}$ pieces Peach
- 65 ml Olive oil
- 2 tablespoon White wine vinegar
- 1 sprig fresh basil
- 1 pinch Salt
- 1 pinch Black pepper

Preparation:

1. Halve the 2 peaches and remove the core.
2. Cut the pulp into pieces.
3. Heat a grill pan and grill the peaches briefly on both sides.
4. Cut the red onion into thin half rings.
5. Roughly chop the pecans.
6. Heat a pan and roast the pecans in it until they are fragrant.
7. Place the arugula on a plate and spread it over the peaches, red onions, blueberries and roasted pecans.
8. Put all the ingredients for the dressing in a blender or food processor and mix to an even dressing.
9. Drizzle the dressing over the salad.

Spinach salad with green asparagus and salmon

Ingredients:

- 2 hands Spinach
- 2 pieces Egg
- 120 g smoked salmon
- 100 g Asparagus tips
- 150 g Cherry tomatoes
- Lemon $^1/_2$ pieces
- 1 teaspoon Olive oil

Preparation:

1. Cook the eggs the way you like them.
2. Heat a pan with a little oil and fry the asparagus tips al dente.
3. Halve cherry tomatoes.
4. Place the spinach on a plate and spread the asparagus tips, cherry tomatoes and smoked salmon on top.
5. Scare, peel and halve the eggs. Add them to the salad.
6. Squeeze the lemon over the lettuce and drizzle some olive oil over it.
7. Season the salad with a little salt and pepper.

Brunoise salad

Ingredients:

- 1 piece Meat tomato
- $1/2$ pieces Zucchini
- $1/2$ pieces Red bell pepper
- $1/2$ pieces yellow bell pepper
- $1/2$ pieces Red onion
- 3 sprigs fresh parsley
- $1/4$ pieces Lemon
- 2 tablespoons Olive oil

Preparation:

1. Finely dice the tomatoes, zucchini, peppers and red onions to get a brunoise.
2. Mix all the cubes in a bowl.
3. Chop parsley and mix in the salad.
4. Squeeze the lemon over the salad and add the olive oil.
5. Season with salt and pepper.

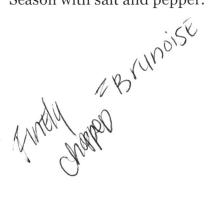

Finely chopped = Brunoise

Broccoli salad

Ingredients:

- 1 piece Broccoli
- $^1/_2$ pieces Red onion
- 100 g Carrot (grated)
- 1 hand Red grapes

Ingredients dressing:

- 2 $^1/_2$ tablespoon Coconut yogurt
- 1 tablespoon Water
- 1 teaspoon Mustard yellow
- 1 pinch Salt

Preparation:

1. Cut the broccoli into small florets and cook al dente for 5 minutes.
2. Cut the red onion into thin half rings.
3. Halve the grapes.
4. Mix coconut yogurt, water and mustard with a pinch of salt to make an even dressing.
5. Drain the broccoli and rinse with ice-cold water to stop the cooking process.
6. Mix the broccoli with the carrot, onion and red grapes in a bowl.
7. Serve the dressing separately on the side.

Ganache squares:

Ingredients:

- 250 ml Coconut milk (can)
- 1 1/2 tablespoon Coconut oil
- 100 g Honey
- 1/2 teaspoon Vanilla extract
- 350 g Pure chocolate (> 70% cocoa)
- 1 pinch Salt
- 2 hands Pecans

Preparation:

1. Place the coconut milk in a saucepan and heat for 5 minutes over medium heat.
2. Add the vanilla extract, coconut oil and honey and cook for 15 minutes. Add a pinch of salt and stir well.
3. Break the chocolate into a bowl and pour the hot coconut milk over it. Keep stirring until all of the chocolate has dissolved in the coconut milk.
4. In the meantime, roughly chop the pecans. Heat a pan without oil and roast the pecans.
5. Stir the pecans through the ganache.
6. Let the ganache cool to room temperature. (You may be able to speed this up by placing the bowl in a bowl of cold water.)
7. Line a baking tin with a sheet of parchment paper. Pour the cooled ganache into it.
8. Place the ganache in the refrigerator for 2 hours to allow it to harden.
9. When the ganache has hardened, you can take it out of the mold and cut it into the desired shape.

Date candy

Ingredients:

- 10 pieces Medjoul dates
- 1 hand Almonds
- 100 g Pure chocolate (> 70% cocoa)
- 2 $1/2$ tablespoon Grated coconut

Preparation:

1. Melt chocolate in a water bath.
2. Roughly chop the almonds.
3. In the meantime, cut the dates lengthways and take out the core.
4. Fill the resulting cavity with the roughly chopped almonds and close the dates again.
5. Place the dates on a sheet of parchment paper and pour the melted chocolate over each date.
6. Sprinkle the grated coconut over the chocolate dates.
7. Place the dates in the fridge so the chocolate can harden.

aleo bars with dates and nuts

Ingredients:

- 180 g Dates
- 60 g Almonds
- 60 g Walnuts
- 50 g Grated coconut
- 1 teaspoon Cinnamon

Preparation:

1. Roughly chop the dates and soak them in warm water for 15 minutes.
2. In the meantime, roughly chop the almonds and walnuts.
3. Drain the dates.
4. Place the dates with the nuts, coconut and cinnamon in the food processor and mix to an even mass. (but not too long, crispy pieces or nuts make it particularly tasty)
5. Roll out the mass on 2 baking trays to form an approx. 1 cm thick rectangle.
6. Cut the rectangle into bars and keep each bar in a piece of parchment paper.

Banana strawberry milkshake:

Ingredients:

- 2 pieces Banana (frozen)
- 1 hand Strawberries (frozen)
- 250 ml Coconut milk (can)

Preparation:

- Peel the bananas, slice them and place them in a bag or on a tray. Put them in the freezer the night before.
- Put all ingredients in the blender and mix to an even milkshake.
- Spread on the glasses.

Buns with chicken and cucumber

Ingredients:

- 12 slices Chicken Breast (Spread)
- 1 piece Cucumber
- 1 piece Red pepper
- 50 g fresh basil
- 3 tablespoons Olive oil
- 3 tablespoons Pine nuts
- Garlic 1 clove

Preparation:

1. Wash the cucumber and cut into thin strips, then cut the peppers into thin strips.
2. Put the basil, olive oil, pine nuts and garlic in a food processor. Stir to an even pesto.
3. Season the pesto and season with salt and pepper if necessary.
4. Place a slice of chicken fillet on a plate, brush with 1 teaspoon of pesto and top the strips with cucumber and peppers.
5. Carefully roll up the chicken fillet to create a nice roll.
6. If necessary, secure the rolls with a cocktail skewer.

Hazelnut balls

Ingredients:

- 130 g Dates
- 140 g Hazelnuts
- 2 tablespoon Cocoa powder
- $^1/_2$ teaspoon Vanilla extract
- 1 teaspoon Honey

Preparation:

1. Put the hazelnuts in a food processor and grind them until you get hazelnut flour (of course you can also use ready-made hazelnut flour).
2. Put the hazelnut flour in a bowl and set aside.
3. Put the dates in the food processor and grind them until you get a ball.
4. Add the hazelnut flour, vanilla extract, cocoa and honey and pulse until you get a nice and even mix.
5. Remove the mixture from the food processor and turn it into beautiful balls.
6. Store the balls in the fridge.

Stuffed eggplants

Ingredients:

- 4 pieces Eggplant
- 3 tablespoons Coconut oil
- 1 piece Onion
- 250 g Ground beef
- 2 cloves Garlic
- 3 pieces Tomatoes
- 1 tablespoon Tomato paste
- 1 hand Capers
- 1 hand fresh basil

Preparation:

1. Finely chop the onion and garlic. Cut the tomatoes into cubes and shred the basil leaves.
2. Bring a large pot of water to a boil, add the eggplants and let it cook for about 5 minutes.
3. Drain, let cool slightly and remove the pulp with a spoon (leave a rim about 1 cm thick around the skin). Cut the pulp finely and set aside.
4. Put the eggplants in a baking dish.
5. Preheat the oven to 175 ° C.
6. Heat 3 tablespoons of coconut oil in a pan on a low flame and glaze the onion.
7. Add the minced meat and garlic and fry until the beef is loose.

8. Add the finely chopped eggplants, tomato pieces, capers, basil and tomato paste and fry them on the pan with the lid for 10 minutes.
9. Season with salt and pepper.
10. Fill the eggplant with the beef mixture and bake in the oven for about 20 minutes.

Chicken teriyaki with cauliflower rice

Ingredients:

- 500 g Chicken breast
- 90 ml Coconut aminos
- 2 tablespoons Coconut blossom sugar
- 1 tablespoon Olive oil
- 1 teaspoon Sesame oil
- 50 g fresh ginger
- 2 cloves Garlic
- 250 g Chinese cabbage
- 1 piece Leek
- 2 pieces Red peppers
- 1 piece Cauliflower (rice)
- 1 piece Onion
- 1 teaspoon Ghee
- 50 g fresh coriander
- 1 piece Lime

Preparation:

1. Cut the chicken into cubes. Mix coconut aminos, coconut blossom sugar, olive oil and sesame oil in a small bowl.
2. Finely chop the ginger and garlic and add to the marinade. Put the chicken in the marinade in the fridge overnight.
3. Roughly cut Chinese cabbage, leek, garlic and paprika and add to the slow cooker. Finally add the marinated chicken and let it cook for about 2 to 4 hours.

4. When the chicken is almost ready, you can cut the cauliflower into small florets. Then put the florets in a food processor and pulse briefly to prepare rice.
5. Finely chop an onion, heat a pan with a teaspoon of ghee and fry the onion. Then add the cauliflower rice and fry briefly.
6. Spread the chicken and cauliflower rice on the plates and garnish with a little chopped coriander and a wedge of lime.

Curry chicken with pumpkin spaghetti

Ingredients:

- 500 g Chicken breast
- 2 teaspoons Chili powder
- 1 piece Onion
- 1 clove Garlic
- 2 teaspoons Ghee
- 3 tablespoon Curry powder
- 500 ml Coconut milk (can)
- 200 g Pineapple
- 200 g Mango
- 1 piece Red pepper
- 1 piece Butternut squash
- 25 g Spring onion
- 25 g fresh coriander

Preparation:

1. Cut the chicken into strips and season with pepper, salt and chili powder. Then put the chicken in the slow cooker.
2. Finely chop the onion and garlic and lightly fry with 2 teaspoons of ghee. Then add the curry powder.
3. Deglaze with the coconut milk after a minute. Add the sauce to the slow cooker along with the pineapple, mango cubes and chopped peppers and let it cook for 2 to 4 hours.

4. Cut the pumpkin into long pieces and make spaghetti of it with a spiralizer (that's not easy, it works better with a carrot).
5. Briefly fry the pumpkin spaghetti in the pan and spread the chicken curry on top.
6. Garnish with thinly sliced spring onions and chopped coriander.

ts:

- 700 g Chicken leg
- 1 tablespoon Olive oil
- 2 pieces Onion
- 4 pieces Carrot
- 2 cloves Garlic
- 8 stems Celery
- 25 g fresh rosemary
- 25 g Fresh thyme
- 25 g fresh parsley

Preparation:

1. Season the chicken with olive oil, pepper and salt and rub it into the meat.
2. Roughly cut onions, carrots, garlic and celery and add to the slow cooker. Place the chicken on top and finally sprinkle a few sprigs of rosemary, thyme and parsley on top. Let it cook for at least four hours.
3. Serve with a delicious salad, enjoy your meal!

Spicy ribs with roasted pumpkin

Ingredients:

- 400 g Spare ribs
- 4 tablespoons Coconut-Aminos
- 2 tablespoons Honey
- 1 tablespoon Olive oil
- 50 g Spring onions
- Garlic 2 cloves
- 1 piece green chili peppers
- 1 piece Onion
- 1 piece Red pepper
- 1 piece Red pepper

For the roasted pumpkin:

- Pumpkin 1 piece
- Coconut oil 1 tablespoon
- Paprika powder 1 tsp

Preparation:

1. Marinate the ribs the day before.
2. Cut the ribs into pieces with four ribs each. Place the coconut aminos, honey and olive oil in a mixing bowl and mix. Chop the spring onions, garlic and green peppers and add them. Spread the ribs on plastic containers and pour the marinade over them. Leave them in the fridge overnight.

3. Cut the onions, peppers and peppers into pieces and put them in the slow cooker. Spread the ribs, including the marinade, and let them cook for at least 4 hours.
4. Preheat the oven to 200 ° C for the pumpkin.
5. Cut the pumpkin into moons and place on a baking sheet lined with parchment paper.
6. Spread a tablespoon of coconut oil on the baking sheet and season with paprika, pepper and salt. Roast the pumpkin in the oven for about 20 minutes and serve with the spare ribs.

Roast beef with grilled vegetables

Ingredients:

- 500 g Roast beef
- 1 clove Garlic (pressed)
- 1 teaspoon fresh rosemary
- 400 g Broccoli
- 200 g Carrot
- 400 g Zucchini
- 4 tablespoons Olive oil

Preparation:

1. Rub the roast beef with freshly ground pepper, salt, garlic and rosemary.
2. Heat a grill pan over high heat and grill the roast beef for about 20 minutes or until the meat shows nice brown marks on all sides.
3. Then wrap in aluminum foil and let it rest for a while.
4. Cut the roast beef into thin slices before serving.
5. Preheat the oven to 205 ° C. Put all the vegetables in a baking dish.
6. Drizzle the vegetables with a little olive oil and season with curry powder and / or chili flakes. Put in the oven and bake for 30 minutes or until the vegetables are done.

Vegan Thai green curry

Ingredients:

- 2 pieces green chillies
- 1 piece Onion
- 1 clove Garlic
- 1 teaspoon fresh ginger (grated)
- 25 g fresh coriander
- 1 teaspoon Ground caraway
- 1 piece Lime (juice)
- 1 teaspoon Coconut oil
- 500 ml Coconut milk
- 1 piece Zucchini
- 1 piece Broccoli
- 1 piece Red pepper

For the cauliflower rice:

- 1 teaspoon Coconut oil
- 1 piece Cauliflower

Preparation:

1. For cauliflower rice, cut the cauliflower into florets and place in the food processor. Pulse briefly until rice has formed. Put aside.
2. Cut the green peppers, onions, garlic, fresh ginger and coriander into large pieces and combine with the caraway seeds and the juice of 1 lime in a food processor or blender and mix to an even paste.

3. Heat a pan over medium heat with a teaspoon of coconut oil and gently fry the pasta. Deglaze with coconut milk and add to the slow cooker.
4. Cut the zucchini into pieces, the broccoli in florets, the peppers into cubes and put in the slow cooker. Simmer for 4 hours.
5. Briefly heat the cauliflower rice in 1 teaspoon of coconut oil, season with a little salt and pepper in a pan over medium heat.

Indian yellow curry

Ingredient:

- 2 pieces Onion
- 1 clove Garlic
- 300 g Chicken breast
- 2 teaspoon Coconut oil
- 1 tablespoon Curry powder
- 1 teaspoonfresh ginger
- 1 teaspoondried turmeric
- Laos 1 tsp
- 500 ml Coconut milk

For the salad:

- 250 g Iceberg lettuce
- $^1/_2$ pieces Cucumber
- 2 pieces Red peppers
- 25 g Dried coriander

Preparation:

1. Heat a saucepan over medium heat and let the coconut oil melt.
2. Finely chop onions and clove of garlic. Put in the pot and add the herbs, deglaze with the coconut milk and stir well.
3. Cut the chicken into cubes and add to the slow cooker along with the curry sauce and let it cook for 4 hours.
4. Cut iceberg lettuce, spread cucumber and bell pepper cubes over it and season with the coriander. Serve the salad with the curry.

Sweet potato hash browns

Ingredients:

- 1 pinch Celtic sea salt
- 1 tablespoon Coconut oil
- 2 pieces Sweet potato
- 2 pieces Red onion
- 2 teaspoons Balsamic vinegar
- 1 piece Apple
- 125 g lean bacon strips

Preparation:

1. Clean the red onions and cut them into half rings.
2. Heat a pan with a little coconut oil over medium heat. Fry the onion until it's almost done. Add the balsamic vinegar and a pinch of salt and cook until the balsamic vinegar has boiled down. Put aside.
3. Peel the sweet potatoes and cut them into approx. 1.5 cm cubes.
4. Heat the coconut oil in a pan and fry the sweet potato cubes for 10 minutes.
5. Add the bacon strips for the last 2 minutes and fry them until you're done.
6. Cut the apple into cubes and add to the sweet potato cubes. Let it roast for a few minutes.
7. Then add the red onion and stir well.
8. Spread the sweet potato hash browns on 2 plates.

Tuna salad in red chicory

Ingredients:

- 4 pieces Red chicory
- 160 g Tuna (tin)
- 1 piece Orange
- 1 tablespoon fresh parsley (finely chopped.)
- 5 pieces Radish
- 1 teaspoon Olive oil
- $1 / 2$ TL Apple cider vinegar

Preparation:

1. Drain the tuna.
2. Cut the orange into wedges and cut them into small pieces.
3. Cut radishes into small pieces.
4. Mix all the ingredients (except the red chicory) in a small bowl. Season with salt and pepper
5. Spread the tuna salad on the red chicory leaves.

Paleolicious smoothie bowl

Ingredients:

- 1 piece Banana (frozen)
- 1 hand Spinach
- $^1/_2$ pieces Mango
- $^1/_2$ pieces Avocado
- 100 ml Almond milk

For garnish:

- Mango$^1/_2$ pieces
- Raspberries1 hand
- Grated coconut1 tablespoon
- Walnuts (roughly chopped)1 tablespoon

Preparation;

1. Put all ingredients in a blender and mix to an even mass.
2. Put the mixture in a bowl and garnish with the remaining ingredients.
3. Of course, you can vary the garnish as you wish.

Granola

Ingredients:

- 160 g Walnuts
- 80 g Almonds
- 80 g Sunflower seeds
- 50 g Grated coconut
- 1 pinch Celtic sea salt
- 1 ¹/₂ tablespoon Coconut oil
- 1 ¹ / ₂ EL Honey

Preparation:

1. Preheat the oven to 150 ° C.
2. Line a baking sheet with parchment paper.
3. Put the nuts, seeds and coconut flakes in a bowl with a pinch of salt and mix well.
4. Add the melted coconut oil and honey and mix well.
5. Spread the mixture on the baking sheet and bake in the middle of the preheated oven for about 20 minutes (until the muesli turns light brown).
6. Let the muesli cool down before removing it from the baking sheet (this creates larger pieces).

Herby Paleo French fries with herbs and avocado dip

Ingredient:

For the Fries:

- $1/2$ pieces Celery
- 150 g Sweet potato
- 1 teaspoon dried oregano
- $1/2$ teaspoon Dried basil
- $1/2$ teaspoon Celtic sea salt
- 1 teaspoon Black pepper
- $1 1/2$ tablespoon Coconut oil (melted)
- Baking paper sheet

For the avocado dip

- 1 piece Avocado
- 4 tablespoons Olive oil
- 1 tablespoon Mustard
- 1 teaspoon Apple cider vinegar
- 1 tablespoon Honey
- 2 cloves Garlic (pressed)
- 1 teaspoon dried oregano

Preparation:

1. Preheat the oven to 205 ° C.
2. Peel the celery and sweet potatoes.
3. Cut the celery and sweet potatoes into (thin) French fries.
4. Place the french fries in a large bowl and mix with the coconut oil and herbs.
5. Shake the bowl a few times so that the fries are covered with a layer of the oil and herb mixture.
6. Place the chips in a layer on a baking sheet lined with baking paper or on a grill rack.
7. Bake for 25-35 minutes (turn over after half the time) until they have a nice golden brown color and are crispy.

For the avocado dip

Puree all ingredients evenly with a hand blender or blender.

Salad with bacon, cranberries and apple

Ingredients:

- 1 hand Arugula
- 4 slices Bacon
- $^1/_2$ pieces Apple
- 2 tablespoon Dried cranberries
- $^1/_2$ pieces Red onion
- $^1/_2$ pieces Red bell pepper
- 1 hand Walnuts

Ingredients dressing:

- 1 teaspoon Mustard yellow
- 1 teaspoon Honey
- 3 tablespoon Olive oil

Preparation:

1. Heat a pan over medium heat and fry the bacon until crispy.
2. Place the bacon on a piece of kitchen roll so that the excess fat is absorbed.
3. Cut half the red onion into thin rings. Cut the bell pepper into small cubes.
4. Cut the apple into four pieces and remove the core. Then cut into thin wedges.
5. Drizzle some lemon juice on the apple wedges so that they do not change color.
6. Roughly chop walnuts.

7. Mix the ingredients for the dressing in a bowl. Season with salt and pepper.
8. Spread the lettuce on a plate / your lunch box and season with red pepper, red onions, apple wedges and walnuts.
9. Sprinkle the bacon over the salad and divide the cranberries.
10. Drizzle the dressing over the salad according to taste.

Strawberry popsicles with chocolate dip

Ingredients

- 125 g Strawberries
- 80 ml Water
- 100 g Pure chocolate (> 70% cocoa)

Preparation:

1. Clean the strawberries and cut them into pieces. Puree the strawberries with the water.
2. If the mixture is not pourable, add some extra water.
3. Pour the mixture into the popsicle mold and put it in a skewer.
4. Place the molds in the freezer so the popsicles can freeze hard.
5. Once the popsicles are frozen hard, you can melt the chocolate in a water bath.
6. Dip the popsicles in the melted chocolate mixture.

Hawaii salad

Ingredients:

- 1 hand Arugula
- $1/2$ pieces Red onion
- 1 piece Winter carrot
- 2 pieces Pineapple slices
- 80 g Diced ham
- 1 pinch Salt
- 1 pinch Black pepper

Preparation:

1. Cut the red onion into thin half rings.
2. Remove the peel and hard core from the pineapple and cut the pulp into thin pieces.
3. Clean the carrot and use a spiralizer to make strings.
4. Mix rocket and carrot in a bowl. Spread this over a plate / lunch box.
5. Spread the red onion, pineapple and diced ham over the rocket.
6. Drizzle the olive oil and balsamic vinegar on the salad to your taste.
7. Season with salt and pepper.

Rainbow salad for lunch

Ingredients:

- 1 hand Salad
- $^1/_2$ pieces Avocado
- 1 piece Egg
- $^1/_4$ pieces green peppers
- $^1/_4$ pieces Red bell pepper
- 2 pieces Tomato
- $^1/_2$ pieces Red onion
- 4 tablespoons Carrot (grated)

Preparation:

1. Boil the egg as you like. (soft / hard / in between)
2. Remove the seeds from the peppers and cut the peppers into thin strips.
3. Cut the tomatoes into small cubes.
4. Cut the red onion into thin half rings.
5. Cut the avocado into thin slices.
6. Cool the egg under running water, peel and cut into slices.
7. Place the salad on a plate / in your lunch box and distribute all the vegetables in colorful rows.
8. If you feel artistic, you can sort the colors from light to dark.
9. Drizzle the vegetables with olive oil and white wine vinegar. Season with salt and pepper.

Strawberry and coconut ice cream

Ingredients:

- 400 ml Coconut milk (can)
- 1 hand Strawberries
- $^1/_2$ pieces Lime
- 3 tablespoons Honey

Preparation:

1. Clean the strawberries and cut them into large pieces.
2. Grate the lime, 1 teaspoon of lime peel is required. Squeeze the lime.
3. Put all ingredients in a blender and puree everything evenly.
4. Pour the mixture into a bowl and put it in the freezer for 1 hour.
5. Take the mixture out of the freezer and put it in the blender. Mix them well again.
6. Pour the mixture back into the bowl and freeze it until it is hard.
7. Before serving; Take it out of the freezer about 10 minutes before scooping out the balls.

Coffee Ice Cream

Ingredients:

- 180 ml Coffee
- 8 pieces Medjoul dates
- 400 ml Coconut milk (can)
- 1 teaspoon Vanilla extract

Preparation:

1. Make sure that the coffee has cooled down before using it.
2. Cut the dates into rough pieces.
3. Place the dates and coffee in a food processor and mix to an even mass.
4. Add coconut milk and vanilla and puree evenly.
5. Pour the mixture into a bowl and put it in the freezer for 1 hour.
6. Take the mixture out of the freezer and scoop it into the blender.
7. Pour it back into the bowl and freeze it until it's hard.
8. When serving; Take it out of the freezer a few minutes before scooping ice cream balls with a spoon.

Banana dessert

Ingredients:

- 2 pieces Banana (ripe)
- 2 tablespoons Pure chocolate (> 70% cocoa)
- 2 tablespoons Almond leaves

Preparation:

1. Chop the chocolate finely, cut the banana lengthwise, but not completely, as the banana must serve as a casing for the chocolate.
2. Slightly slide on the banana, spread the finely chopped chocolate and almonds over the bananas.
3. Fold a kind of boat out of the aluminum foil that supports the banana well, with the cut in the banana facing up.
4. Place the two packets on the grill and grill them for about 4 minutes until the skin is dark.

Salad with roasted carrots

Ingredients:

- 1 hand mixed salad
- 500 g Carrot
- 1 piece Orange
- 100 g Pecans
- $^1/_2$ teaspoon dried thyme
- 1 tablespoon Honey
- 1 tablespoon Olive oil
- 1 pinch Salt
- 1 pinch Black pepper

Preparation:

1. Peel the carrots and cut the green. Cut them in half lengthways.
2. Cook the carrots al dente for 5 minutes and drain well.
3. Peel the orange and cut it into pieces.
4. Roughly chop the pecans and briefly fry them in a pan without oil.
5. Cut the spring onions into thin rings.
6. Place the carrots in a bowl with 1 tablespoon of olive oil, a pinch of salt and pepper and the thyme.
7. Roast the carrots briefly on the grill or in a grill pan. Until they have nice grill marks.
8. Mix the salad with carrots and honey and put on a plate.
9. Spread the orange slices and pecans over the salad.

'th capers and lemon

- 2 pieces Salmon fillet
- 1 tablespoon Coconut oil
- 2 tablespoon Capers
- $^1/_2$ pieces

Preparation:

1. Cut the lemon into thin slices.
2. Take an aluminum tray or piece of aluminum foil that is folded in half.
3. First lay out 4 slices of lemon and spread the capers on them.
4. Place the salmon on the capers. Then put a lemon wedge on the salmon.
5. Fry the salmon on the grill (with aluminum dish / foil).
6. Season with salt and pepper just before serving.

Pasta salad

Ingredients:

- 125 g green asparagus
- 1 hand Cherry tomatoes
- $^1/_2$ pieces yellow bell pepper
- $^1/_2$ pieces Red bell pepper
- 125 g Sesame fusilli

Ingredients dressing:

- 3 tablespoon Olive oil
- 1 tablespoon Red wine vinegar
- 1 teaspoon dried oregano

Preparation:

1. Cook the sesame fusilli as indicated on the package.
2. After cooking the pasta, drain with cold water.
3. Slice the green asparagus into pieces.
4. Heat a grill pan and grill the asparagus al dente.
5. Cut the cherry tomatoes into pieces; some in halves and some in quarters, this gives the salad a nice playful effect.
6. Cut the two half peppers into long thin strips.
7. Mix the pasta, asparagus, tomatoes and peppers in a large bowl.
8. Mix the ingredients for the dressing in a small bowl.
9. Stir the dressing through the pasta salad.

Pine and sunflower seed rolls

Ingredients:

- 120 g Tapioca flour
- 1 teaspoon Celtic sea salt
- 4 tablespoon Coconut flour
- 120 ml Olive oil
- 120 ml Water (warm)
- 1 piece Egg (beaten)
- 150 g Pine nuts (roasted)
- 150 g Sunflower seeds (roasted)
- Baking paper sheet

Preparation:

1. Preheat the oven to 160 ° C.
2. Put the pine nuts and sunflower seeds in a small bowl and set aside.
3. Mix the tapioca with the salt and tablespoons of coconut flour in a large bowl. Pour the olive oil and warm water into the mixture.
4. Add the egg and mix until you get an even batter. If the dough is too thin, add 1 tablespoon of coconut flour at a time until it has the desired consistency.
5. Wait a few minutes between each addition of the flour so that it can absorb the moisture. The dough should be soft and sticky.
6. With a wet tablespoon, take tablespoons of batter to make a roll. Put some tapioca flour on your hands so the dough

doesn't stick. Fold the dough with your fingertips instead of rolling it in your palms.

7. Place the roll in the bowl of pine nuts and sunflower seeds and roll it around until covered.
8. Line a baking sheet with parchment paper. Place the buns on the baking sheet.
9. Bake in the preheated oven for 35 minutes and serve warm.

Spiced burger

Ingredients:

- Ground beef 250 g
- 1 clove Garlic
- 1 teaspoondried oregano
- 1 teaspoon Paprika powder
- $1/2$ TL Caraway ground

Ingredients toppings:

- 4 pieces Mushrooms
- 1 piece Little Gem
- $1/4$ pieces Zucchini
- $1/2$ pieces Red onion
- 1 piece Tomato

Preparation:

1. Squeeze the clove of garlic.
2. Mix all the ingredients for the burgers in a bowl. Divide the mixture into two halves and crush the halves into hamburgers.
3. Place the burgers on a plate and put in the fridge for a while.
4. Cut the zucchini diagonally into 1 cm slices.
5. Cut the red onion into half rings. Cut the tomato into thin slices and cut the leaves of the Little Gem salad.
6. Grill the hamburgers on the grill until they're done.
7. Place the mushrooms next to the burgers and grill on both sides until cooked but firm.

8. Place the zucchini slices next to it and grill briefly.
9. Now it's time to build the burger!
10. Place 2 mushrooms on a plate, then stack the lettuce, a few slices of zucchini and tomatoes. Then put the burger on top and finally add the red onion.

Chicken skewers with cashew sauce

Ingredients:

- 2 pieces Chicken legs
- 1 $^1/_2$ EL Coconut amino
- 1 clove Garlic
- 1 tablespoon Sesame seeds
- 1 tablespoon Olive oil
- $^1/_2$ pieces Spring onions
- 4 pieces Toothpicks

Ingredients cashew sauce:

- 75 g unsalted cashew nuts
- 75 ml Coconut milk
- 1 $^1/_2$ EL Coconut amino
- 1 clove Garlic

Preparation:

1. Cut the chicken legs into cubes and put them in a bowl.
2. Add coconut aminos and olive oil and press the clove of garlic into the mixture.
3. Stir with a spoon and let marinate for about 30 minutes.
4. In the meantime, put a few long wooden skewers in water.
5. Put the chicken cubes on the skewers.
6. Put the ingredients for the cashew sauce in a food processor and grind until you get a smooth sauce.
7. Place the sauce in a saucepan and heat slowly until hot. (slow is very important, otherwise the sauce can separate)
8. Cut the spring onions into rings.
9. Grill the chicken skewers on the grill, garnish with the spring onions and sesame seeds. Serve with the warm cashew sauce.

Vegetable skewers

Ingredients:

- $1/2$ pieces Eggplant
- $1/2$ pieces Zucchini
- $1/2$ pieces yellow bell pepper
- 4 pieces Cherry tomatoes
- 1 clove Garlic
- 3 tablespoons Olive oil
- $1\ 1/2$ EL Balsamic vinegar
- 4 pieces Toothpicks

Preparation:

1. Place the skewers in a bowl or bowl of water about half an hour before you start cooking
2. Cut the aubergine, zucchini and bell pepper into 8 pieces.
3. Put all the vegetables on the skewers.
4. Squeeze the garlic and mix with the oil and balsamic vinegar.
5. Drizzle the dressing over the skewers.
6. Grill the vegetables on the grill for about 5 minutes.
7. Drizzle a little more dressing on the skewers before serving.

Pork chops with orange and mustard glaze

Ingredients:

- 2 pieces Rib cutlet
- 1 piece Orange
- 1 tablespoon Mustard yellow
- 1 tablespoon Olive oil
- 2 sprigs fresh rosemary

Preparation:

1. Put the pork chops in a bowl.
2. Squeeze the orange and put it in a bowl with the mustard and olive oil.
3. Take the rosemary leaves and add them to the orange mixture.
4. Beat well for a minute and then pour the mixture over the pork chops.
5. Leave on for at least 45 minutes.
6. Grill the pork chops on the grill.

Grilled sweet potato with coriander dressing

Ingredients:

- 2 pieces Sweet potato
- 1 tablespoon Coconut oil

Ingredients dressing:

- 1 hand fresh coriander
- 2 $^1/_2$ tablespoon Olive oil (mild)
- 1 tablespoon Natural vinegar
- $^1/_2$ pieces Red pepper

Preparation:

Wash the sweet potato and cut lengthways into slices about 1 cm thick.

Place the slices in a bowl and pour coconut oil over them. Add a little salt and mix well.

Grill the sweet potato on the grill until it is done.

In the meantime, do the dressing; Put all the ingredients in the food processor and mix to an even dressing.

Serve the sweet potato with the dressing.

Conclusion

Sirtfoods are the pioneering methods to activate our Sirtuin genes in the best possible way. These are the miracle foods that are particularly rich in natural natural chemicals, the so-called polyphenols, that our sirtuin genes can activate by turning on. Essentially, they mimic the effects of fasting and exercise and offer remarkable benefits by helping the body better control blood sugar, burn fat, build muscle, and strengthen health and memory.

Because plants are stationary, they have developed a sophisticated stress response system and produce polyphenols to adapt to the challenges of their environment. When we consume these plants, we also consume these polyphenol nutrients. Their effect is profound: they activate our own innate stress response pathways.

While all plants have stress response systems, only a few have evolved to produce remarkable amounts of sirtuin-activating polyphenols. These plants are sirt foods. Your discovery means that instead of strict fasting plans or strenuous exercise programs, there is now a revolutionary new way to activate your sirtuin genes: a diet rich in sirt foods. The best thing is that the diet is to put food on your plate and not lose weight.

There is growing evidence that sirtuin activators have various health benefits, strengthen muscles, and suppress appetite. These include improved memory, better control of blood sugar levels by the body, and the elimination of damage caused by free radical molecules that accumulate in cells and can lead to cancer and other diseases.

"There are many observations about the beneficial effects of using sirtuin and food activators to reduce the risk of chronic disease," said Professor Frank Hu, nutritionist and epidemiologist at Harvard University, in a recent report. Article in the magazine on advances in nutrition. A sirt food diet is particularly suitable as an anti-aging diet.

Although sirtuin activators are present throughout the plant kingdom, only certain types of fruits and vegetables are large enough to be considered sirt-food. Examples are green tea, cocoa powder, turmeric with Indian spices, kale, onions and parsley.

Many fruits and vegetables on display in supermarkets such as tomatoes, avocados, bananas, lettuce, kiwis, carrots, and cucumbers actually contain small activators of sirtuins. However, this does not mean that they are not worth eating since they offer many other benefits.

The good thing about a sirt diet is that it is much more flexible than other diets. You can just eat healthy and add sirt foods. Or you could have concentrated them. If you add sirt foods, the 5: 2 diet can add more calories on low-calorie days.

One notable finding from a sirt diet study is that the participants lost considerable weight without losing muscle. In fact, it was common for participants to actually develop muscles, which resulted in a lighter, firmer appearance. It's the good thing about sirt food. They activate fat burning, but also promote growth, maintenance and repair of muscles. This is in sharp contrast to other diets where weight loss usually results from both fat and muscle, with muscle loss slowing metabolism and making weight gain more likely.